Herbal Highs and Aphrodisiacs

Adam Gottlieb &

Mary Jane Superweed

Ronin Publishing

Berkeley, CA

Herbal Highs and Aphrodisiacs

Adam Gottlieb &
Mary Jane Superweed

Herbal Highs & Aphrodisiacs

Copyright 2019 by Ronin Publishing
ISBN: 9781579512859 Pbook
ISBN: 9781579512873 Ebook

Published by
Ronin Publishing, Inc.
PO Box 3436
Oakland, CA 94609
www.roninpub.com

Production:

 Manuscript creaton: Beverly A. Potter.
 Book Design: Beverly A. Potter.
 Cover Design: Brian Groppe
 Content Creation: John Mann

Library of Congress Control Number: 2019949277

Distributed to the book trade by PGW/Ingram.

This book was compiled from material in *Herbal Highs*, copyright 1970 by SKS/TCA; *Home Grown Highs*, copyright 1972 by SKS/TCA; and *Herbal Aphrodisiacs*, copyright 1971 by SKS/TCA—all of which were authored by John Mann, aka Mary Jane Superweed.

Table of Contents
Herbal Highs and Aphrodisiacs

Table of Contents continued

PART ONE:
Herbal Highs and Aphrodisiacs

The purpose of this book is to introduce the reader to herbs, cacti, mushrooms and other members of the vegetable kingdom that can get you high. It covers important information, such as correct dosage, methods of use, effects, after-effects and chemical nature of the psychoactive substances involved. Most of the plants mentioned are quite potent, legal and readily available in field, forest, or garden. However, the author, editor and publisher of this guide do not encourage the use of any of these substances.

Some of the botanicals discussed have potential dangers, which are clearly pointed out without exaggeration. One man's treat can be another man's poison. So if readers decide to experiment with psychedelic herbs it is best to proceed with caution. Persons in poor health—especially those with diabetes, epilepsy, heart, liver or blood pressure problems—are advised not to use these or any other psychedelic substances with-out consulting their physician. Neither should one go cheerfully about the countryside and garden munching or toking on all the pretty flowers in hopes of finding a new high. Many common plants, such as water hemlock and oleander, are deadly poisons.

Readers who elect to experiment with psychedelic herbs should check their health safety and proceed with caution.

The pictures of plants shown in this manual serve as aids, but not as a final and positive identification. Those who wish to be sure that a plant is what they think it is must learn to use a botanical key. These may be found in a public library. There is no telling where and when any of these herbs may be outlawed. Readers should check the laws of their state and community.

WILD CUCUMBER
(Echinocystis lobata)

In the early 1960s several children in Ojai, California, began conversing with nonexistent persons and showing other

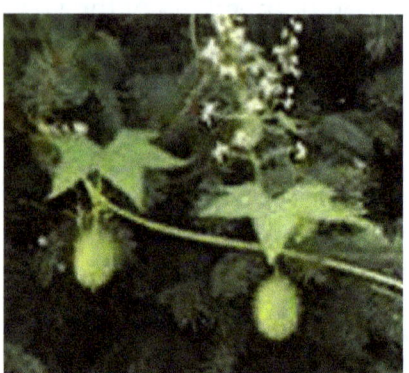

Wild Cucumber

symptoms of severe hallucination. Later it was learned that they had been nibbling on the seeds of wild cucumbers. This low crawling vine of the melon family can be found growing among thickets along the coastal slopes of California, Washington and Oregon, as well as in many other places throughout the U.S. It has greenish-white flowers and a spiny, green, oblong fruit containing four large seeds.

There is no information available as to the exact chemical nature of the hallucinogens in wild cucumber—possibly lysergic acid amides, but they are most effective when the seed is not quite ripe, around middle or late spring. One seed is considered to be a good experimental starting dose. Birds eat the seed for food without any harmful results, but since its chemistry is still unknown so are its possible dangers. The trip lasts for eight to ten hours and no harmful side effects have been noted.

LOBELIA
(*Lobelia inflata*)

The leaves of lobelia (also called "Indian Tobacco") have an acrid tobacco-like taste. For this reason they are often smoked as a cigarette substitute by people trying to break the nicotine habit. When smoked as a joint, retaining the smoke in the lungs, lobelia has mildly euphoric marijuana-like qualities while conferring to the mind a great sense of clarity.

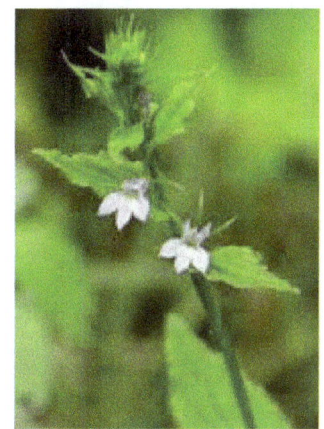

Lobelia

Taken as a tea its effect is even more pronounced. It has the unique ability of acting simultaneously as both a relaxant and a stimulant, which results in a dynamically altered mental state. Two heaping tablespoons of the leaves and stems are simmered in a pint of water. The tea causes a prickly sensation in the mouth and throat, which some people find unpleasant. To circumvent this one may prepare twice the dose and, after straining, reduce the tea by boiling until only a dark, gummy residue remains. This can be mixed with a pinch of the dried leaves to give it substance and put into a large 000 size capsule.

The active principle of lobelia is a crystalline alkaloid called *alpha-lobeline*. It is officially classified as a poison because it has a tendency in large doses to induce vomiting. Lobelia has been used for centuries in herbal medicine and has no real toxic history. The tea or capsules is taken on an empty stomach.

KAVA-KAVA
(*Piper methysticum*)

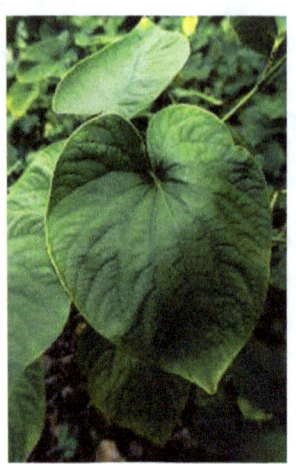

Kava-Kava

Throughout the islands of the South Pacific for many centuries the root of a shrub belonging to the pepper family has been used as a narcotic, mood elevator and ceremonial beverage. When the Presbyterian missionaries forbade its use it was largely replaced by alcohol. It is, however, still used on many of the islands.

Most scientific authorities agree that kava is a potent but uniquely harmless narcotic. The most common way to use kava is to shave away the outer bark from the root until the pale pink or yellow inner rhizome is all that remains.

This is cut into small pieces and two good mouthfuls of these are thoroughly chewed and swallowed. In a few of the islands another method is used which produces the most potent effect:

(I) Three heaping tablespoons of the inner rhizome of fresh kava root are shaved off—6 tbsp. if using dried kava.

(2) The shavings are boiled for five minutes with one pint of water in a non-metal or stainless steel container with the top covered.

{3) The liquid is strained off and put it in a clear glass container.

(4) The mixture is put in the refrigerator for 24 hours.—In the islands it is sometimes left for several weeks in cool streams. It is now ready to sip slowly. A peaceful and elated feeling in about twenty minutes with

heightened perceptions. Very sensitive people have been known to hallucinate beautiful sounds and colors. When taking kava it is considered best to avoid complicated matters, activity, wordy conversation and alcohol.

With fresh roots a trip lasts about six hours; with dried roots much less. There are no unpleasant long- or short-range effects from its use. Kava is not habit forming. Islanders drink it about twice a week. Its psychedelic qualities are due to C6-aryl substituted alpha pyrones: kawin, dihydrokawin, methysticin, dihydromethysticin, yangonin and desmethoxyyangonin.

HAWAIIAN BABY WOOD ROSE
(*Argyreia nervosa*)

The immature seeds of Hawaiian baby wood rose contain lysergic acid amides, and other alkaloids. Dried wood rose stalks with seed pod clusters are rather decorative and can be purchased inexpensively at many florists. Four to eight seeds is the usual dose. The seeds are remove from the pod. The fuzz which coats the seed is removed either with a toothbrush or by inserting a long needle into the seed and thoroughly singeing the outer coating in a candle flame for several seconds. The seeds can then be thoroughly chewed and swallowed or pulverized in a pepper grinder and put into large 000 size gelatin capsules.

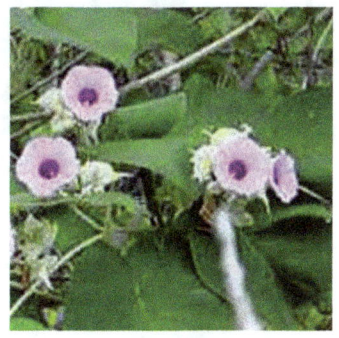

Hawaiian Baby Wood Rose

Wood rose seeds are best taken on an empty stomach in a peaceful environment. The trip is generally best enjoyed when alone or with someone with whom one has an undisturbing and quiet relationship. Wordy people can be incredibly irritating. It takes about an hour to come on. At first there is a feeling of weakness and lethargy. Those with a sensitive stomach may get nauseous for about fifteen minutes. Experienced trippers suggest sipping a little warm water or mint tea and vomiting if necessary. Dramamine pills—available at any drug store without prescription—may also help. After this has passed one generally feels very relaxed and peaceful yet very aware. This state of bliss lasts for about three or four hours and is followed by a gradual descent to normality accompanied with feeling unusually relaxed and mellow for several days.

MORNING GLORY
(Ipomoea purpurea)

The seeds of certain varieties of morning glories contain substances similar to LSD. Between five and ten grams is a good dose. Rather than buying seed packages, it is more economical to purchase a five-pound sack from a feed and seed store. Also packaged seeds are often treated with

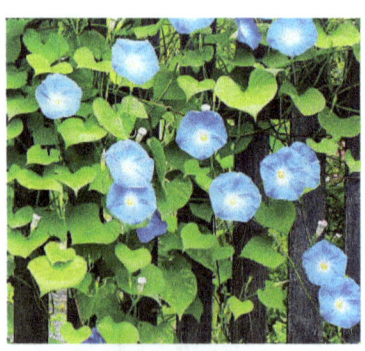

Morning Glory

chemical that may be poinsonous. Treated seeds can be cleansed by soaking them in warm water for twenty minutes. The most hallucinogenic varietes are Pearly Gates, Flying Saucers, Wedding Bells and Heavenly Blue. Some "glory heads" prefer Pearly Gates to Heavenly Blue because they are reputed to give the most dramatic effects.

If simply eatting the seeds, they pass through the body undigested without getting stoned. The best method of ingesting morning glory seeds is one used by the Mexican Indians: the seeds are run several times through a pepper grinder. Then after soaking the seed mash in a glass of water for about eight hours, the liquid is strained through a cloth and drunk.

EXTRACTING LYSERGIC ACID AMIDES FROM MORNING GLORY AND HAWAIIAN WOOD ROSE SEEDS

Yield is 1 strong dose per 30 grams of morning glory seeds or per 15 seeds of Hawaiian wood rose.

1. Grind 100 grams of seeds in an osterizer, pepper or coffee grinder.
2. Soak in 120 cc petroleum for 2 days.
3. Filter solution through a paper filter.
4. Discard liquid.
5. Allow mash to dry completely.
6. Soak dried mash in 100 cc methyl alcohol for 2 days.
7. Filter solution, label liquid "Solution A" and save.
8. Resoak mash in 100 cc methyl alcohol for 2days.
9. Filter and discard mash, add liquid to solution A.
10. Pour solution into a large flat tray and let evapo rate in a well-ventulated shady space.

A yellow gum remains when alohol is gone, which may be scraped up and rolled with enough flour to remove tackiness and stuffed into capsules. Gum that remians stuck to tray may be dissolved with water and drunk.

The LSD-like substances contained in morning glory are: *d*-lysergic and *d*-isolysergic acid amides, lysergol, chanoclavine, elymoclavine and ergonovine. They are about one-tenth the potency of LSD. Three hundred seeds are about equal to 300 micrograms of LSD-25. Pure LSD-25 can be synthesized from these amides.

Two other types of morning glory which are even more potent than *I. purpurea* come from Mexico. These are *I. violacea*, known there as "badoh negro" and *Rivea corymbosa* or "oluliuque".

HYDRANGEA
(Hydrangea paniculata grandiflora)   ,

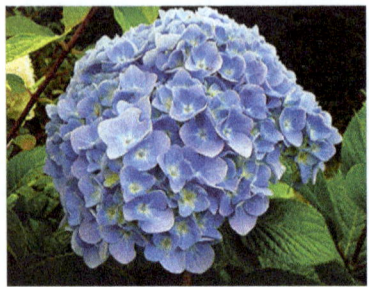

Hydrangea

The leaves of one of America favorite garden shrubs, when dried and smoked, can get a person quite stoned. But this practice can be dangerous. Hydrangea leaves contain a chemical that belongs to the cyanide family. The high derived from this is an example of subtoxic inebriation, in which there is a fairly narrow margin between pleasurable and toxic doses. The greatest dangers are either from smoking too much or too often. In the latter case the body may not get rid of the poison as quickly as the user accumulates it.

HELIOTROPE
(Valeriana officinalis)

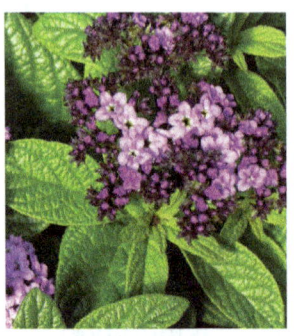

Heliotrope

The roots and rhizomes of this well-known garden plant contain a very potent tranquilizer called valeric acid. Unfortunately they also have a very potent odor. The tea, however, has at least a tolerable flavor. Boil 1/2 oz. for five minutes in a pint of water with the pot covered. If you do not wish to test your tolerance with the taste of the tea, strain this brew and reduce its volume by evaporation till a gummy residue remains. This can be rolled with a pinch of flour and stuffed into a large gelatin capsule.

PEYOTE
(*Lophophora williamsii*)

This small button-like cactus is a native of Mexico and the American Southwest. Its major hallucinogenic alkaloid is mescaline, but it does contain several other active substances including lophophorine, a convulsant; pcllotine, a sedative; and anhalonidine, a central nervous system stimulant. Three to ten fresh or dried peyote buttons are chewed and swallowed after the white fur has been removed. The first effects that occur in thirty or forty minutes, are perspiration, shivers, nausea and possible vomiting. This may sound terrible, but a subtle alteration of consciousness has already begun, which usually makes these inconvenient symptoms seem not particularly disturbing.

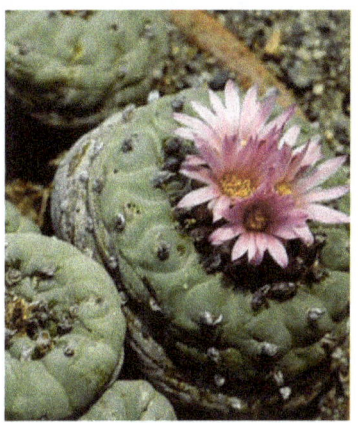

Peyote

In less than an hour these effects will have passed and the psychedelic characteristics of the cactus will be active. These include altered mental state, intensified audio and visual perceptions, and hallucination of colorful patterns especially while eyes are closed or room is darkened. The entire experience lasts about six hours. Because peyote has an overwhelmingly bitter taste and a tendency to produce nausea numerous methods of ingestion have been devised which circumvent the problem. Here are several:

> Mescaline is the major hallucinogenic alkaloid in peyote.

(1) Run the buttons through a pepper grinder several times and put the ground material in large 000 gelatin capsules.

(2) Drinking grapefruit juice while consuming the peyote can neutralize the bitterness.

(3) Ground-up buttons can be boiled in water for five hours. Then the resulting tea can be strained off. By further boiling, the volume of tea is reduced to a thick syrup which upon cooling is a semi-soft gum, which can be put into gelatin capsules.

The shock of peyote alkaloids on the system can be lessened by dividing the full dose into two half doses, which are taken thirty minutes apart.

Legal Status

Recreational use of peyote is prohibited in all of the states and territories and by federal law. Recreational use can bring large fines and even jail time. Use of peyote for non-religious purposes is also against the law in the United States.

While once illegal, the United States now exempts ceremonial use of peyote as legal—but restricted to the Native American Church and does not extend to other Native American groups that use peyote in religious ceremonies. Consequentally, a number of religious peyote growers and users have been prosecuted under local laws.

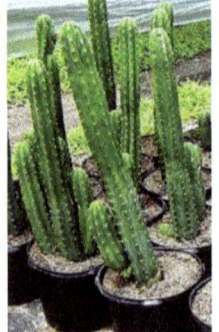

San Pedro

SAN PEDRO
(*Trichocereus pachanoi*)

This large columnal cactus is native to Peru, but is available in the United States. Its main active ingredient is mescaline. It is, however, much larger than the little peyote buttons, which are the best known source of that alkaloid,

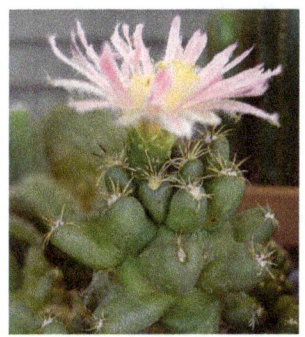

Dona Ana

so many turn-ons can be enjoyed from a single plant. The correct dose is about is about three times the peyote dose.

DONA ANA
(Coryphantha macromeris)

Dona Ana is a small cactus from northern Mexico. Its major active ingredient is macromerine, which is a phenethylamine hallucinogen chemically related to mescaline. Macromerine is only about one-fifth the potency of mescaline so it is necessary to take two or three grams of the pure extracted alkaloid or five times as much, in weight of the cactus, as with peyote.

CALIFORNIA POPPY
(Eschscholtzia califomica)

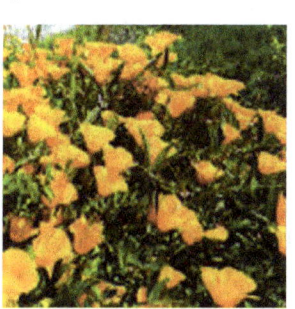

California Poppy

When pot is scarce many West Coast people smoke the leaves and orange petals of this common wildflower. It is not an opium poppy but it does contain some unknown substance, which offers a mild high lasting about 30 minutes. Although there are no narcotics laws against its use, it is the official flower of the State of California and is under protection. Persons caught picking or mutilating this poppy are subject to fine.

MESCAL BEANS
(Sophora secundiflora)

This shrub of the American Southwest and northern Mexico bears dark red beans which are hallucinogenic. Their psychoactive nature is due to the presence of a

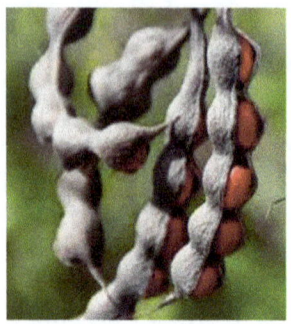

Mescal Beans

toxic pyridine called cytisine. It has powerful psychedelic virtues. However, as a warning, it can cause nausea and convulsions, and in excessive doses it has been known to cause an occasional death from respiratory failure.

This bean was once used in ritual by the Indians of the plains and northern Mexico, but it was later replaced by a safer sacrament, peyote. The mescal bean should not be confused with mescaline or with mescal, an alcoholic beverage made from maguey plants. Experimentation with the bean is not recommended.

COLORINES
(*Rhynchosia phaseloides*)

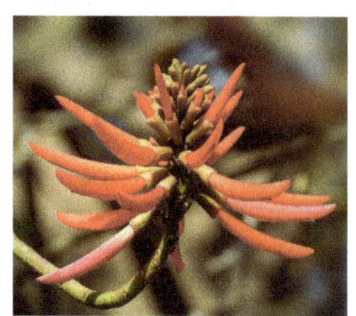

Colorines

These red beans and often the black ones of *R. pyramidalis* are similar to mescal beans in both hallucinogenic qualities and dangers. These characteristics are caused by a toxic indole or isoquinol. The Indians sold these beans as ornamental beads at the marketplace in Oaxaca and usually warned the customer of the danger of consuming them.

WILD LETTUCE
(*Lactuca virosa et al.*)

This species of wild, prickly lettuce and, to varying degrees, most other types of wild and cultivated lettuce including common head lettuce—*L. sativa capita*—contain lactucarium, contain lactucarium, a bitter alkaloid resembling opium in physical properties. This substance, also called "lettuce opium", was formerly used as a sedative, but now it is, at least in the pharmaceutical world, largely replaced by opium derivatives and synthetics. Informed chemists, however, who have had difficulty in procuring actual opium, have learned to extract its sister substance from various members of the lettuce family.

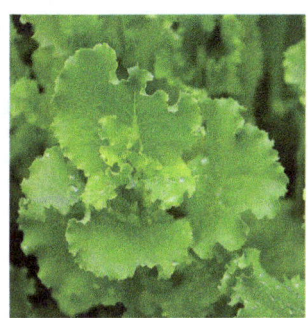

Wild Lettuce

To accumulate lactucarium the entire wild lettuce plant and/or the bitter hearts and roots of market lettuce is run through an electric vegetable juicer. As much juice as possible—at least a pint—is extracted. This liquid is poured into a porcelain or glass bowl and set it in the hot

sunlight or under heat lamps until the water content has evaporated leaving a greenish-brown gummy residue, which is scraped from the bowl with a kitchen knife and used like opium. Direct flame should never be applied to opium or lactucarium as this destroys most of the qualities.

A small piece of lettuce opium can be placed in a tiny brass pipe bowl and, with the pipe pointed slightly downward, while heating the bowl, until the "opium" bubbles, giving off a white smoke or vapor, which can be inhaled for an enjoyable high.

A small piece of lettuce opium can be placed in the tiny brass pipe bowl and, with the pipe pointed slightly downward so that the gum will not go up the stem, heated over a candle, alcohol lamp, bunsen-burner or wooden match. The flame should barely lick over the top of the bowl until the "opium" begins to bubble, giving off a white smoke or vapor. This vapor can be inhaled into the lungs for about thirty seconds. Lactucarium is not as potent as the very highest quality opium but many are surprised at its virtues. The name "head" lettuce may acquire a new and punful meaning in the psychedelic subculture.

DAMIANA
(*Turnera diffusa*)

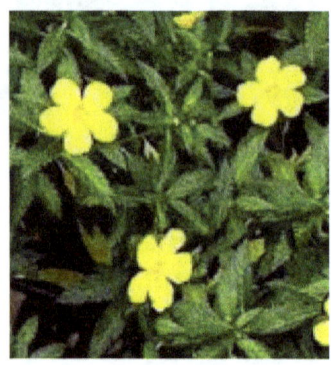

Damiana

Tea made from the leaves of this tropical American shrub—also found in Texas and California—has been long known as a mild aphrodisiac and tonic for the reproductive organs. Although it is a little harsh on the throat, smoking will trigger a high, if it is smoked in a water pipe the harshness is satisfactorily reduced.

Fortunately it does not take much for a turn on. One pipe load is generally enough. Its effect is about that of medium quality grass and lasts about an hour to an hour and a half. It gets one even more stoned when drinking the tea while smoking it. One tablespoon of damiana leaves can be simmered in a pint of water for three minutes. Its taste is not bad, but it is a little on the bitter side so some honey is often added.

NUTMEG
(*Myristica fragrans*)

This well-known commercial spice is ground from the fruit of a tree grown in the East and West Indies. Its mind-altering properties have been recognized for centuries in India, and it has often been used by prisoners in the United States as a substitute for other psychedelies and euphoriants which were not available.

Doses exceeding one teaspoonful take effect within two to five hours, producing time-space distortions, feelings of unreality and sometimes visual hallucinations. Although some people thoroughly enjoy the trip others have suffered ill feelings, headache, rapid heartbeat and dizziness. The active constituents of nutmeg are found in the aromatic oil. These arc elemicin and myristicin, both of which arephenylpropenes similar in structure to mescaline, and the synthetics MDA and TMA. They are also present in mace, another common spice. Because different lots of nutmeg and mace contain widely varying amounts of the substances results of experiments are often inconsistent.

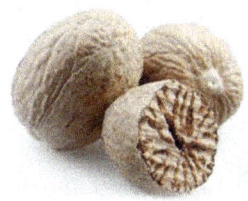

Nutmeg

If one or two teaspoons of nutmeg produce no effect, dosage can be increased up to about one gram for every two pounds of body weight; in other words no more than one 1-3/8 oz. for an average adult male. The peak experience lasts from five to eight hours and is usually followed by drowsiness and sleep with lethargic feelings lasting throughout the next day.

CAUTION

Epileptics should not experiment with large doses of nutmeg.

FLY AGARIC
(*Amanita muscaria*)

This poisonous, hallucinogenic mushroom is found in Europe, Asia and North America. For many centuries it has been used as an intoxicant by the primitive people of northeastern Asia. One large mushroom of the light red variety is dried n the open air or in smoke and then eaten.

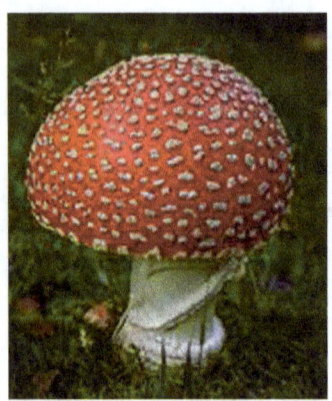

Fly Agaric

The effect begins one or two hours after ingestion with trembling and twitching followed by numbness of the limbs. Then for a while good humor and contentment pervade. After that hallucinations and foolish behavior occur. Sometimes the user becomes red-faced and violent or suffers vomiting and diarrhea. Prolonged used of the mushroom can be mentally debilitating.

The psychoactive principles of *Amanita muscaria* are muscazon, ibotcnic acid and also muscimol, which has the unusual characteristic of passing unaltered through the kidneys. In Siberia, where the mushroom is costly, it has been rumored that the poor often drink the urine of the rich to get high. When at wild gatherings the initial intoxication begins to dwindle, people drink their own and each other's urine to get a second high.

Unappealing though it may be to most of us, imbibing this psychoactive waste product is the satest way to ingest *Amanita muscaria* because the poisons muscarine and muscaridine have been metabolized and are not excreted. Small agarics with numerous white warts are more potent and more toxic than the pale red and less spotted variety. A North American species, *Amanita pantherina*—panther caps, is more deadly than *Amanita muscaria*.

CAUTION

The greatest problem with *Amanita muscaria* is that the margin between an effective and a lethal dosage is narrow.

One of the greatest problems in using these mushrooms is that the margin between effective and lethal dosage is narrow. The correct amount varies with the individual so that one man's dose could be another man's doom. Atropine is the standard antidote for agaric poisoning. It is understandable when a poor Siberian gambles with poisonous mushrooms since they are his only temporary escape from a grim environment. But it is foolish to toy with these dangers when there is such a wide selection of relatively safe psychedelic botanicals at our command.

KOLA NUTS
(*Cola nitida*)

Kola nuts possess more stimulating effects than can be accounted for by the amount of caffeine present in them. Like coffee beans they contain about 2 percent of the drug. The added punch is credited to the essential oil. Africans believe that kola is an aphrodisiac for men and promotes conception in women.

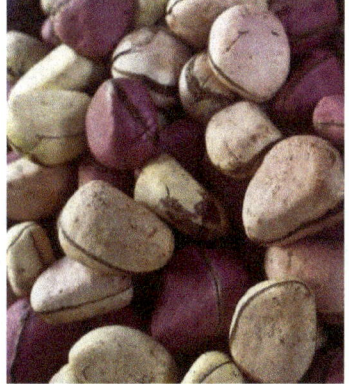

Kola Nuts

Western science revealed that it is an economizer of the muscular and nervous systems and that it augments the combusion of fats and carbohydrates in the body while reducing the combustion of nitrogen and phosphorus. Two nuts is a good starting dose. These may be chewed and swallowed or ground up and brewed as a beverage. One or two teaspoonsful of honey brings out the delicious lavor of the kola oil.

SYRIAN RUE
(*Peganum harmala*)

This 12-16 inch herb, also called African rue, is found in India, the eastern Mediterranean countries and on the treeless plains of Spain. Its seeds and root contain the phenolic

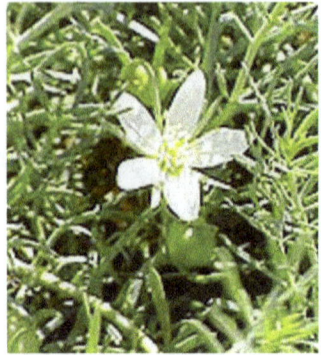

Syrian Rue

alkaloids harmine, harmaline and harmalol, which are also the active ingredients of the Peruvian vine from which yage is made. These substances are powerful stimulants and are capable of inciting wild visions. The usual amount of pure alkaloids taken to produce such results is 300 mg. or more.

This is about the same dosage as mescaline, but the effects of harmine and harmaline are far more striking. People traveling in the Mediterranean countries, where Syrian rue is sold commercially as a spice, have occasionally brought back a few of the seeds and raised them in greenhouses. The plant enjoys a lot of sunlight. The seeds are sometimes used in the U.S. and in Europe as a stimulant and to get rid of worms. Since it is such a dramatic stimulant experimenters should be cautious with dosages. Ten grams or so of the seeds or root should suffice to start. If this is not enough the amount can be safely increased gradually.

Syrian rue is a member of the caltrop family, and is not related to any of the American or North European rues. Recently a substance called *6-methoxytetra-hydroharman*, which is closely related to the active ingredients in yage and Syrian rue and about one-third the potency of harmine and harmaline, has been isolated from the hormone secreted by the pineal gland—third eye—oman. This fragment of information serves to remind us that the real source of natural and legal turn-ons exists within ourselves.

CAMPHOR
(*Cinnamomum Camphora*)

Camphor eating was at one time a great fad in some circles. It acts as a reflex stimulant by irritating the nerve

CAUTION

Do not confuse genuine camphor with paradichlorobenzine moth flakes, which are highly toxic.

endings. One gram produces a pleasant, warm, tickling sensation on the skin, ecstatic mental excitation and an impulse to move about. Two grams brings on thought floods, ego loss, vomiting, amnesia, delirium and convulsions, all lasting for about three hours with possible recurrence several hours later. Camphor tincture or powedered camphor has occasionally been added to grass and smoked. This gives the grass a slightly stimulating effect.

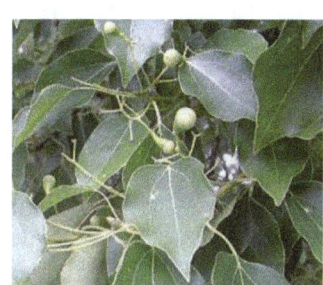

Camphor

YOHIMBE
(*Corynatithe yohimbe*)

This tree grows in the Bantu country of tropical West Africa. It is a member of the Rubiaceae family, a group of medicinal plants which are rich in alkaloids. The bark of the yohimbe tree contains the powerful psychoactive alkaloid yohimbine.

In small doses yohimbine acts as a hypotensive, that is, it lowers tension and blood pressure. In slightly larger amounts is has strong psychedelic effects. The bark also contains several other alkaloids including yohimbiline, which, when reacted with hydrochloric acid, forms a potent aphrodisiac substance called quebrachine—*yohimbiline hydrochloride.*

Taking a yohimbe trip involves adding six to ten teaspoons of

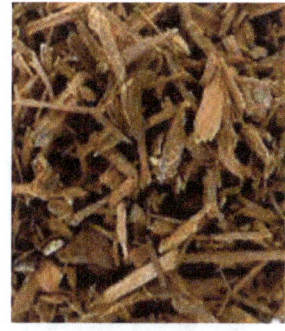

Yohimbe Bark

shaved yohimbe bark to a pint of boiling water.Heat is
then lowered as solution simmers for five minutes with
pot dovered, then strained and drunk as a tea. This makes
about two cups and is the recommended dosage for one
person. The tea should be taken on an empty stomach
and consumed within fifteen minutes. After about half an
hour the tripper begins to feel the first effects of the drug:
a lethargic weakness of the limbs and a vague restlessness
similar to the initial effects of LSD. Chills and shivers may
also be felt, accompanied in some instances by very slight
dizziness and nausea—not as strong as is often the case
with peyote. After about fifteen minutes most of these feelings will have passed and the psychedelic characteristics of
the drug begin to take effect. Depending, of course, on the
individual these may be a relaxed and somewhat inebri-
ated mental and physical feeling with intensified visual
responses and possible color flashes.

The trip lasts from three to four hours and leaves no
unusual after-effects other than a pleasantly relaxed feeling
and occasionally a running nose which should persist for no
more than a few hours. There are no indications of addiction or harmful long-range effects from the occasional use of
yohimbe.

ARECA NUTS
(*Areca catechu*)

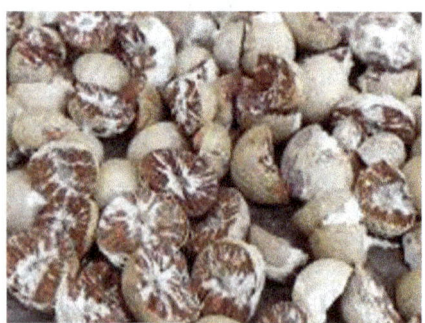

In 1930 Louis Lewin
estimated that there were
about 200,000,000 betel
nut chewers in the world-
The betel nut—more
correctly called the betel
morsel-consists of a piece
of areca nut from the areca
palm tree —*Areca catechu*,

Areca Nuts

a betel leaf—*Piper chavica betel,* some catechu gum from a Malaysian acacia tree—*Acacia catechu*—and a pinch of burnt lime. The exciting effect of the betel morsel on the nervous system is mainly due to the oily volatile arecoline contained in the areca nut. The lime helps to release the arecoline.

CAUTION

Excessive use of betel morsels can cause a dark red staining of the mouth and teeth.

Arecoline causes increased salivation, excitation of the central nervous system, more rapid respiration and decrease of the work load on the heart. If the areca nut is unripe it will contain more arecoline and may cause dizziness and inebriation. Unfortunately arecoline can also irritate the mucous membranes of sensitive individuals and produce liquid stools. Catechol, the oil of catechu—also called catechin—is a white crystalline phenol alcohol which is distilled or extracted from the acacia. The betel morsel or areca nut is held under the tongue and sucked on like a piece of hard candy.

HOPS
(*Humulus lupulus*)

Hops is a possible altrnative to marijuana. The female hops plant contains a yellow powder which is chemically related to cannabis resin—hashish. An old-time cure for insomnia was to sleep on a pillow stuffed with hops. Unfortunately, in some highly sensitive individuals this can cause dizziness, mental stupor and possible jaundice symptoms.

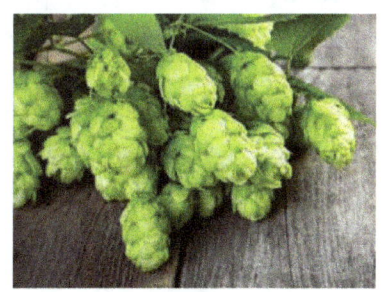

Hops

A safe method of using hops as a sedative is as follows: Steep 1 oz. of hops in a pint of boiling water. Allow to stand for two hours and strain. One tablespoonsful is taken before each meal and before retiring. A more interesting aspect of hops is that it is marijuana's closest relative. Therefore it can be grafted to marijuana roots.

This will produce hops which are rich in cannabinol resins. Used like grass they get the smoker as high as grass. It is impossible to say what the legal status of cannabinated hops may be, because it has not been tested in the courts. There are many reasons why it might be impossible for the authorities prosecute such a case. Furthermore it is unlikely that narcotic agents would ever discover hopped-up hops since in appearance the plant does not resemble marijuana.

Salvia Divmorum

PIPIZINTZINTLI
(*Salvia divmorum*)

This broadleaf sage of the mint family is native to southern Mexico, but it can grow in the U.S. It is used by the Mazatec Indians when psilocyb mushrooms are out of season. Its effect is similar to that of the sacred mushroom but shorter lasting and less overwhelming. Fifty or more leaves arc thoroughly crushed in a bowl. A pint of lukewarm water is poured over them and they are allowed to steep for a few hours. Then the liquid is drunk and the leaf mash can be chewed and swallowed.

Visual hallucinations of dancing colors and elaborate designs may be experienced as well as telepathic and clairvoyant insights. Attempts to analyze the plant's chemistry have been unsuccessful, probably because its components are unstable. The answer may add valuable information to psychopharmacology. But until its chemistry is known it is difficult to pass laws against its use.

COLEUS
(*Coleus blumei and C. pumila*)

These two species of coleus and all of their garden varieties have strong psychoactive qualities. Although originally from Southeast Asia, they are now familiar in the United States and Mexico as both indoor and outdoor plants. They have a long history in folk medicine in the Old World, and have been used for many years by the Mazatec Indians of Southern Mexico in the same manner and for much the same effect as Salvia divmorum.

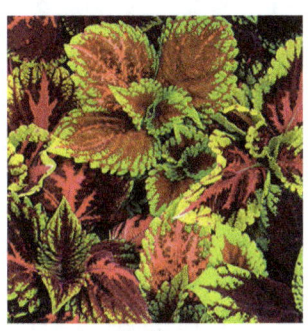

Coleus

About fifty of the brightly coloredleaves arc either chewed and swallowed, or crushed and steeped in water which is later drunk. (See description of preparation under "Pipizintzintli" above.) Like Salvia divinorum, coleus is a member of the mint family, so the psychoactive chemistry of the two plants is probably identical or at least similar. Potted coleus plants are available at any nursery or the seeds may be purchased from most packaged seed racks. Considering the number of leaves required, it is far more economical to grow your own from the seeds.

JIMSON WEED
(*Datura stramonium*)

This plant, also called thorn apple, devils apple or stinkweed, grows wild in many places including India, Mexico and the United States. It belongs to the potato family—*Solanaccae*—and has dark green leaves and a

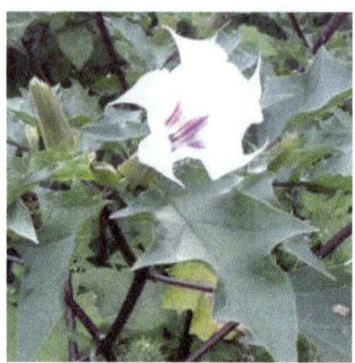

Jimson Weed

large bell-shaped flower. The entire plant is rich in several medicinal alkaloids: atropine, scopolamine, mandragorinc and hyoscyaminc. The leaves of datura are often smoked to relieve asthma symptoms. In India two or three seeds and some leaves are added to ganga—*cannabis*—for an extra kick. It can, however, cause blacking out and severe head aches.

The brujos—sorcerers—of Mexico claim that the leaves and stems of the local species, *D. tneteloides*, which they call devil's weed, are for medicine, and the root and seeds for divinatory and hallucinogenic purposes. But the flowers, they say, will drive a person mad.

The Yaqui Indian brujos extract a drink from datura by crushing the root in water. Because the process is very involved it will not be discussed here. The reader is referred to *The Teachings of Don Juan: A Yaqui Way of Knowledge* by Carlos Castaneda. The effects from datura are pressure on the head, visual distortion, hallucinations and sleep.

Smoking the leaves produces euphoria. Although its influence is not so intense as that from drinking the root extract, which if done to excess can bring on amnesia, confusion and sluggish thinking. Datura and other Solanaceae contain

CAUTION

The brujos maintain that psychological dependence on Jimson Weed is a very real danger.

tropeins which are bad for the heart. Datura is not physically addicting but it can be very dangerous. While one builds up a tolerance for the narcotic and hallucinogenic substnaces in this herb and comes to require larger dosages to produce the desired effect, one does not build a tolerance for the tropeins and eventually they will do severe damage to the heart. And even the brujos maintain that psychological dependence on the drug is a very real danger.

DEADLY NIGHTSHADE
(*Atropa belladonna*)

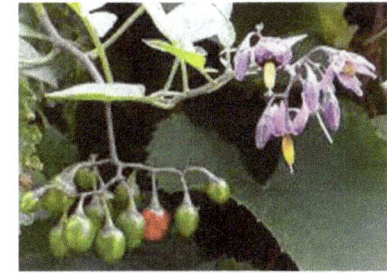

Deadly Nightshade

This plant is the source of the drug belladonna, which is actually a combination of atropine, scopolamine and hyoscyamine. The drug gets its name from the Italian bella donna, "beautiful lady," because since Roman times women on the Italic Peninsula used it to dilate the pupils and make the eyes appear brighter.

The drug also has a long history in witchcraft, medicine, and murder; and has been sold as LSD by unscrupulous racketeers. It is strongly hallucinogenic, but it can have many unpleasant side effects such as headache, intestinal cramps, loss of appetite and mental stupor, if the dose is too large. The plant grows wild in many places throughout North America.

HENBANE
(*Hyoscyamus niger*)

The leaves, seeds and rhizomes of this common plant are chemically similar to datura and are very rich in hyoscyamine, a drug which is similar to atropine, but twice as powerful in its effects on the peripheral nervous system. It causes fantastic

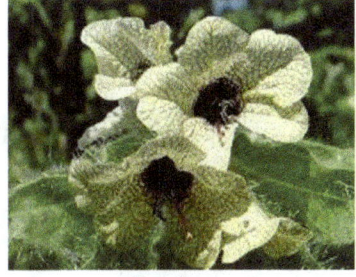

Henbane

visual hallucinations, and has been used by occultists to conjure demons.

Its dangers are similar to those of datura. Even the sorcerers of ancient Europe agreed that excessive use of henbane can cause permanent insanity. The leaves of one variety of hyoscyamus are smoked in India and Africa for their inebriating effect.

MANDRAKE
(*Mandragora officinarium*)

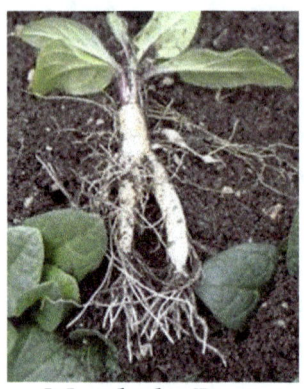

Mandrake Root

Not to be confused with the New World mandrake or May apple—*Podophyllum peltatum*, this plant with its supposedly human-shaped root—actually the root looks like a parsnip—is the basis of many legends. It was a standard ingredient of witches' brews. The chemistry of mandrake is similar to that of datura and it is exceptionally rich in mandragorine, a powerful narcotic and hypnotic. Any of the dangers which have been expressed regarding datura are equally true of mandrake.

CATNIP
(*Nepeta cataria*)

Because of its apparently happy influence on cats many humans have tried to devise a method of using this herb of the mint family which would give them a similar high. The tea is useful in folk medicine, but has no appreciable

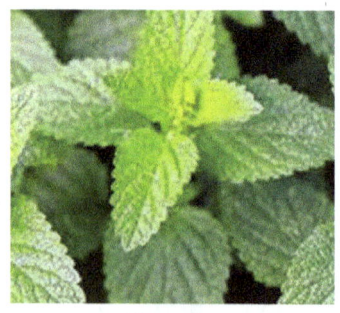

Catnip

mind-altering properties. Smoked as a joint or in a pipe its effects are similar to a mild marijuana high. When it is mixed half and half with tobacco and used as a cigarette its influence is more intense and longer-lasting.

Another successful method is to spray tobacco with the liquid extract available from pet shops in a spray can or to collect a small amount of extract in a glass and inject it into a cigarette. The active chemistry of catnip is in the volatile oil, but it is not yet certain which of the several oily constituents is responsible. Catnip burns rapidly and since it is weaker than pot larger quantities are required.

SCOTCH BROOM

(Cytisus scoparius or Sarathamnus scoparius)

Heads seeking new highs or unable to score any pot sometimes harvest the yellow flowers of scotch broom, store them in a jar for two weeks or until they become moldy, dry them and smoke them as a joint.

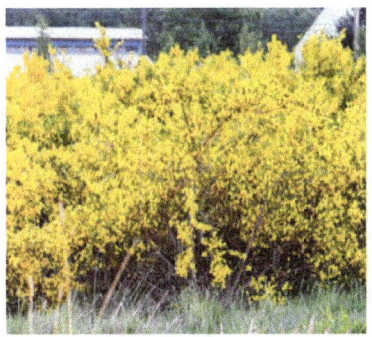

Scotch Broom

The plant, a native of Western Europe, is cultivated here but has escaped from gardens and is often found growing on hill slopes and in vacant lots. Its intoxicating properties have been known for many centuries because sheep which have nibbled on it are sometimes found in a state of stupor.

When Ingested the plant acts on the heart in much the same manner as red foxglove, the source of the cardiac stimulant digitalis.

CAUTION

When ingested the Scotch Broom acts on the heart to cause excitation followed by unconsciousness or stupor.

It causes excitation followed by unconsciousness or stupor. When smoked its effect is not so extreme—mostly stimulation and euphoria. Because of its effect on the heart it can be dangerous, and too much of it is definitely injurious.

MEXICAN CALEA
(*Galea zacatechicha*)

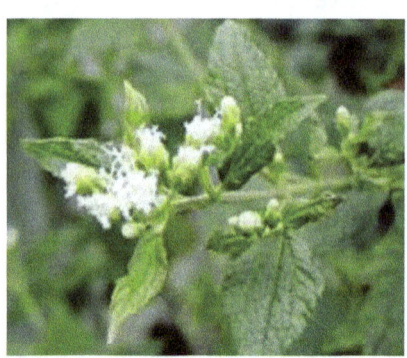

Mexican Calea

This shrub of the Compositae family is said to be the most recent natural psychedelic discovery of science. It has, of course, been known and used by the Chontal Indians of Oaxaca for many centuries. They call it Thle-pela-kano, which means "the leaf of God," and employ it as a tea to clarify the senses.

Two tablespoonfuls are steeped for five minutes in a pint of boiled water, strained, and sipped slowly. The dried leaves can be purchased inexpensively at the marketplace in Oaxaca. Not much is known about its chemistry, but it appears to have no adverse side effects.

OTHER HIGHS

Adventurous heads have come up with several interesting substitutes for grass and the other illegal highs. Smoking the dried scrapings from the inside of banana skins—mellow yellow—was a popular fad during the late sixties. Some experts believe that combustion converts some of the banana's chemistry into bufotenine—a DMT-like chemical, but since it takes three or four joints to get even a mild buzz there is much doubt as to the usefulness of this substance.

The Jackson illusion pepper—named after its discoverer—consists of a rotten green pepper with a cigarette in one end and a hole in the opposite end through which the entire contraption is smoked. It is said to produce colorful and elaborate hallucinations. Some call it a hoax, others credit the effect to deep inhalation of the tobacco smoke, but several scientists have stated that certain alkaloids in the rotten pepper are converted to bufotenine when contacted by the cigarette smoke and the heat. *Caution:* Tobacco is dangerous, addicting and deceptively legal. Some claim that they can get heavily stoned from smoking ZNA, a foul-tasting blend of dill weed and monosodium glutamate.

Others say they have had a good trip smoking petunia leaves and tomato leaves. This is possible since the petunia and tomato belong to the same family as tobacco and jimson weed. Peanut skins are supposed to be another smokable turn-on, but actually they taste unpleasant and have a very dull effect. Niacin—one of the B vitamins—has a pronounced result when taken in doses of about 100 mg. It causes prickly feelings of the skin and a strange, dizzy feeling for about twenty minutes. Powdered cinnamon can be smoked with parsley or mint flakes. It produces warm, tingling sensations all over the body followed by a stimulated and transparently aware sort of high. It seems to act as a mild irritant to the nerve endings similarly to camphor.

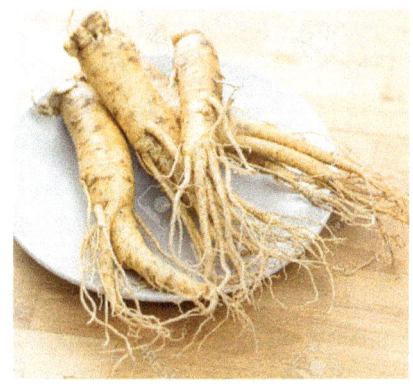

Many Americans as well as Orientals swear that ginseng root has both stimulating and rejuvenating powers. Unfortunately most of the ginseng sold in this country—*Panax quinquefolium*—is not the same

Korean Ginseng

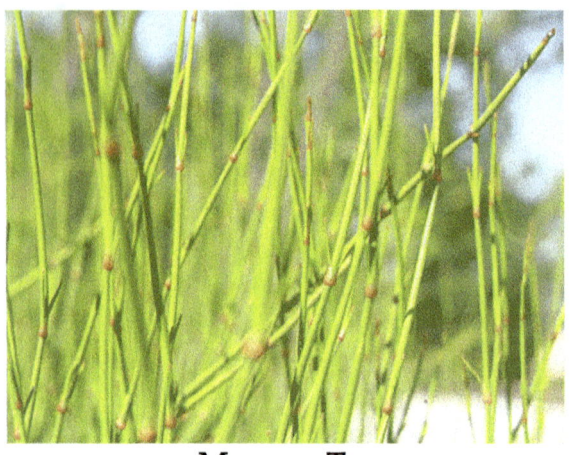

Mormon Tea

as the Oriental kind—*P. schinseng*, which is sold in some Chinatown sections under the name Korean Ginseng.

Seeds of *Strychnos nux-vomica*, the source of strychnine, have occasionally been ingested in minute quantities for their stimulating effect upon the spinal cord and cerebrum. In very exacting doses it has also been found to enhance the learning processes. *aution:* the margin between useful and dangerous (usually lethal) doses is very narrow. Wormwood—*Artemisia absinthium*—yields a dark, green-brown, bitter essential oil with strong narcotic properties.

Although absinthe, an alcoholic beverage containing this oil, is illegal in this country, the herb itself is legal. The narcotic oil can be extracted with water or alcohol. Excessive use of this drug is said to be debilitating, however. Mormon tea—*Ephedra nevadensis*, a plant found in the semi-desertareas of the central United States, contains the well-known crystalline alkaloid ephedrine, a sympathomimetic which acts on the autonomic nervous system.

Copious quantities of the tea have a peculiarly stimulating effect. Mexican locoweed—*Astragalus mollissimus*—is found in the prairie lands of New Mexico, Texas, Colorado, Montana and the Dakotas. Cattle which graze upon it display symptoms of temporary insanity. Prairie folk do not recommend it for humans. *Rauwolfia serpentina*, also called Indian snakeroot, but not at all similar to American snakeroot, is the source of the powerful tranquilizer rescrpinc. It is usually sold only by prescription.

Other useful tranquilizing herbs are: musk root—*ferula sumbul*—2 to 4 tbps. simmered 5 minutes in 1 pint of water (fresh root preferred. Skullcap—*Scutellaria lateriflora*—1/2 oz. steep in 1 pt. boiled water and let stand 1 hour. Horsetail—*Bquisetum arvense*—steep 1/2 oz. in 1 pt. water—fresh plant preferred. German or Hungarian Chamomile (*Matricaria chamomilla*) 1/2 oz. in 1 pt. boiled water; steep and let

sit 2 hours. Asafetida gum (*Ferula asafoetida*) 1/2 tsp. in warm water. Passionflower (*Passiflora incarnata*) 1/2 oz. steeped in 1 pt. boiled water.

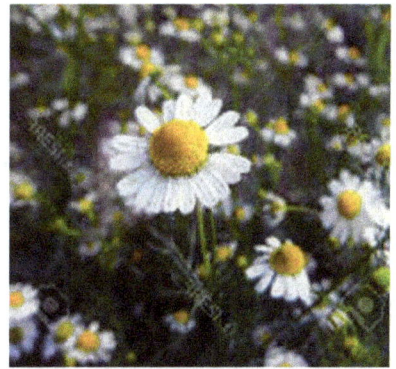

Hungarian Chamomile

Strained passionflower leaves may be smoked for a mild (but very relaxing) high or as a tobacco substitute by unfortunates who are trying to recover from nicotine addiction. Its odor, when burning, is almost identical to that of marijuana. Defense attorneys could make much use of it in pot cases in which the police made their arrests on the basis of smelling marijuana.

PART TWO:
Home Grown Highs

Because of an increasing difficulty in procuring reliable organic psychedelics may people grow their own. When governement operation intercept went into effect marijuana became so scarce and expensive that manypeople were forced to follow in the footsteps of George Washington, Thomas Jefferson and other Great Americans by becoming gentlemen hemp farmers.

We at Stone Kingdom have been proud to serve our fellow Americans—and fellow Humans around the world—by publishing agricultural information on the cultivation of cannabis. Today marijuana plants flourish by the millions in secluded fields, greenhouses, hydroponic tanks, flower pots, window boxes and illuminated closets across the nation.

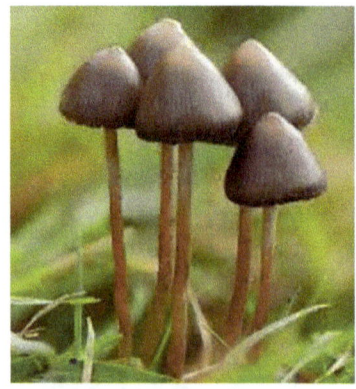

Psilocybe Mushrooms

There has been a complaint, however, about the shortage of good quality mescaline, psilocybin and other natural psychedelics. Many are screaming out against the frightful substances which some street dealers are trying to pass as organic highs. The cry was heard and Stone Kingdom offers this book as an answer.

CULTIVATING RAPID-GROWING, HIGH-YIELD
PSILOCYBE MUSHROOMS

Many people have inquired about the cultivation of the psychedelic mushroom, *Psilocybe mexicana.* They usually ask how to grow the mushroom and where to acquire the spores. Although the cultivation of psilocybe mushrooms requires care and attention it is not as difficult as one might imagine. Also it takes far less time to raise them than any other psychoactive plant. A popular misconception is that it is necessary to cultivate the fungi to the extent of producing catpophores, the familiar umbrella-shaped fruiting bodies of the plant that house the spores.

Actually the greater part of the plant lies beneath the ground. It is a fibrous network of living matter known as the mycelium or mycelial mat. Whereas the carpophores only appear briefly during certain seasons, the mycelium is present most of the time and can be grown on culture media all year round. The mycelium contains as much psilocybin as the carpophore itself and can be cultivated in a matter of days.

The problem of finding psilocybe spores should not hinder one. Although *P. mexicana* is usually found only near the remote mountain village of Huautla de Jimenez in the state of Oaxaca in southern Mexico, there are at least fifteen varieties of mushrooms rich in psilocybin and psilocin which can be found in most parts of the United States and parts of Canada. Nor does one have to acquire spores from these to raise our mycelial cul-

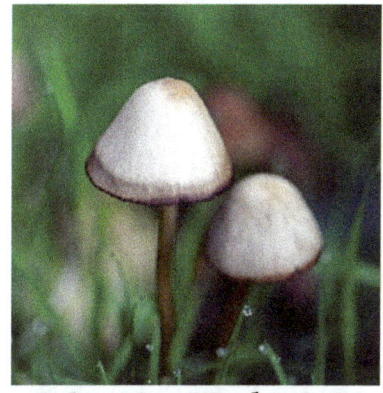

Cultivating Mushrooms

tures. Any portion of the carpophores or mycelium may be used to propagate new plants.

FINDING THE MUSHROOM

The following species have been tested and found to contain psychoactive indole compounds *psilocin and/or psilocybin; Psibcybe baeocystis, P. caerulescens, P.* caeru*lipes, P. cubensis var. cyanescens, P. cyanescens, P. pelli cubsa, P. quebecensis, P. semilanceata, P. sitvatica, P. strictipes, Conocybe cyanopes, Pholiotina cyanopoda, Copehndia cyanescens, Panaeolus foenisecci, P. subbalteatus.*

These are not to be confused with the often dangerous and sometimes deadly amanita mushrooms which may possess traces of psilocybin but mostly contain a different group of alkaloids. The species listed here are psychoactively potent but not physically harmful. Those who enjoy psychedelics have a pleasant time with them. A possible exception to this statement may be applicable to the species *Psibcybe baeocystis*. It has been reported that in 1960 a six-year-old boy died from eating a large number of baeocystis mushrooms.

The poisoning was apparently due to the presence of two alkaloids: baeocystin and nor-baeocystin. These alkaloids have not been found in any of the other species listed here and occur only in small harmless quantities in the baeocystis mushroom. Adults have taken normal doses of this species without any ill effects. Caution is advised, however, when using crude alkaloidal extractions of psilocybin from *P. baeocystis* until more has been learned about the species.

Incorrect identification of mushrooms can be anything from disappointing to fatal. Because of this we will not attempt to outline identification tech-

CAUTION

Incorrect identification of mushrooms can be anything from disappointing to fatal.

niques in this article. Instead we recommend that the reader obtain a good textbook on the subjectpreferably one with clear color photographs. Also one should learn to use botanical identification keys. These contain exacting and detailed descriptions of all parts of each species. If a plant does not conform precisely in every respect to the key, using it may be a risk.

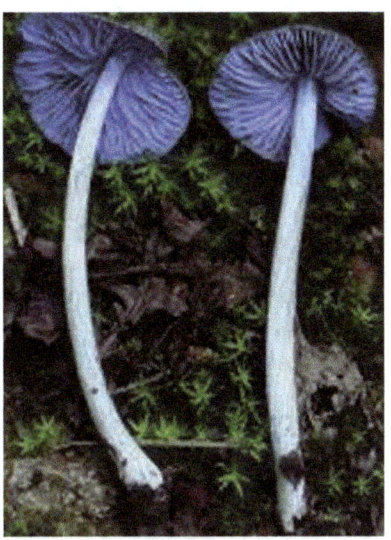

Bluish Mushrooms

Fortunately there is a test that will determine whether a mushroom contains alkaloids of the psilocin/psilocybingroup: After thorough and satisfactory identification has been completed scratch the surface of the mushroom. Within several minutes to several hours the injury will turn blue or bluish green if it is a psilocybin-bearing mushroom. This color change is due to a chemical reaction between the psilocybin, various enzymes in the mushroom, and atmospheric oxygen. To save time in the field while hunting the mushroom, hunters bring a small bottle containing a freshly mixed solution of one part Metol—a developing agent found in any photo supply store—also known as Elon and 20 parts distilled water—by weight. After being convinced that the mushroom in question fulfills the proper description in every detail the specimen can be plucked by grasping the stem-not the cap.

The entire carpophore is cleaned with a Q-tip or wad of cotton-wool.

Inoculation is a most exacting part of mushroom cultivation.

Caps are severed from stem and allowed to fall into a clear plastic baggie. The stem is cut into two pieces, putting each half in a separate baggie. Metol solutionting is added to one, both baggies are sealed with wire tape ties. Both stem pieces are crushed inside the baggies. The metol-treated piece will turn bluish violet in less than 30 minutes if identification is correct.

If it does then observe the untreated stem piece. This should turn blue or bluish green after several hours. If it does not, discard your specimen. Be sure to label all three parts of the specimen. This test works on all psilocybin-bearing species with the possible exception of Panaeolus foenisecci.

CULTIVATING THE MYCELIUM

The following formula is designed for maximum mycelial growth and maximum psilocybin yield. It is based on the findings of Catalfolmo and Tyler at the Drug Plant Laboratory of the College of Pharmacy at the University of Washington in Seattle:

Three hundred grams of unpeeled potatoes are washed and sliced 1/8 inch thick, and wash again until water is clear. After the water is drained. they are rinse once with distilled water and drain again and cooked in one liter distilled water until tender, using stainless steel or pyrex—never iron or aluminum. Next it is filtered through clean flannel cloth into a jar and rinseed two more times with distilled water, filtering each time into jar. Then potatoes are discarded. When necessary distilled water is added to make one liter.

The resulting liquid is poured into a pot and brought to a boil, then the heat is immediately turned off heat and 15 grams agar is added, stirring until completely dissolved, taking care that it does not boil over. Then 10 grams dextrose is added. Note the dextrose should be pure, not commercial because many commercially processed forms of dextrose contain enough lead to inhibit growth. Next 1/2 gram yeast extract, 1 gram ammonium succinate, 1 gram potassium acid phosphate—KH_2PO_4, 100 mg. thiamine HC1, 1/4 oz. TMS are added, adjusting to pH 5.5 with hydrochloric acid.

For best results it is recommended that the following be prepared in advance: a trace mineral stock solution—TMS—containing 8 mg. ammonium molybdenate—$(NH4)6Mo7O24*4H2O$, 50 mg. zinc sulphate $ZnSO4*7H2O$, 50 mg. manganese chloride $MnCl2*4H2O$, 350 mg. iron sulphate $FeSO4*7H2O$, 75 mg.

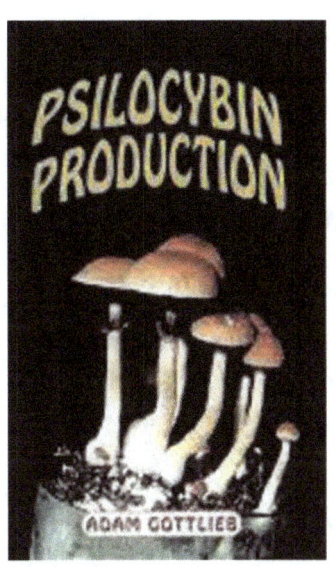

How to grow psilocybin mushrooms

copper sulphate $CuSO4*5H2O$.75 mg. magnesium sulphate $MgSO4*7H2O$, and distilled water to make 1 liter. Some cultivators like to add 2 mg. aureomycin and 30 mg. streptomycin at this point to prevent bacterial contamination.

While liquid is still hot 30 ml. is poured into each 125 ml. Erlenmeyer flask and capped with a two-hole rubber stopper. The stopper is covered with a large wad of sterile cotton wool and cotton pulled down about neck of flask and binded with tape wire ties.

While liquid is still hot it is poured into clear baby bottles, which come in sets of nine or ten with steam sterilizer. One liter of medium will fill a set of bottles. If a ten set they are filled to 100 ml. mark; if a nine set they are fill to 110 ml. then immediately capped upon filling.

Caps are modified by cutting tips of nipples to leave an opening 1/4 inch in diameter. Clean sterile cotton-wool is stuffed into cap from bottom of cap and pulled about 1/2" through the top. Excess cotton is trimmed at top to 1/4" length. Bottles tilted at 17° angle and liquid is allowed to cool and agar to gel. Generally a stand that will hold bottles at this angle is constructed. Bottles are steralized for 30 minutes at 212° in steamer. Process is repeated the next day and again on third day. Bottles are then returned to slant stand while still hot and allow to cool. Bottles are now ready for inoculation. Because these bottles are kept tilted during incubation they are called slants.

INOCULATION

Inoculation is a most exacting part of mushroom cultivation. Great care must be taken to insure that no other fungi or bacteria overrun the culture. The instructions given next must be followed precisely if contamination it so be avoided. All parts of the mushroom including pieces of the mycelium may be used to propagate new cultures, but, when starting with specimens gathered in the field, the part least likely to be bacterially contaminated is the inner flesh of the caps.

Immediately before commencing work everything is washed, including the work table and surrounding area with a strong disinfectant such as Lysol and a disinfectant sprayed in the room. Simple clothing is worn, such as a clean, short-sleeved T-shirt. Wearing a cloth or disposable paper-cloth surgeon's mask over your mouth and nose is recommended because our breath contains millions of bacteria. For added protection it is advisable to gargle first with antiseptic

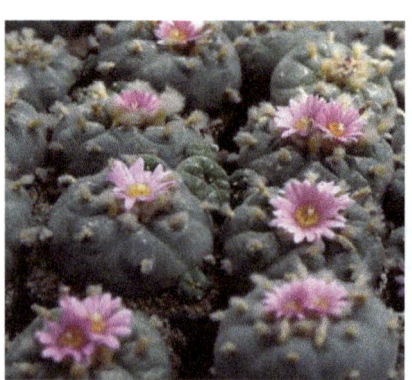

Growing peyote

mouthwash. One's hair should be covered with a shower cap or surgeon's cap. One's arms, hands and fingernails should be scrubbed with strong disinfectant soap. Drafts shuld not be allowed to enter the room by closing windows and stuffing door jams.

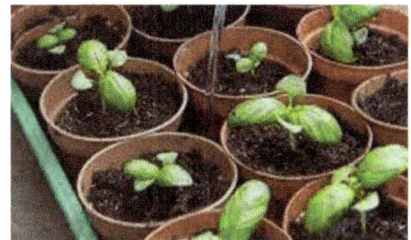

Growing cacti

Swift movements that might cause drafts are avoided. The room must be simple, uncluttered and dust-free. A cardboard or canvas or sheet metal hood that open only at the front help to keep dust, spores and other undesirable material from falling on the work space. Animals are not allowed in the room as well as no more people than are absolutely necessary to perform the work. One should not lean over the work, which may enable microorganisms to drop into it. Everything shuld be orderly and kept within easy reach.

Specimen cap is removed from the baggie and placed with gills down upon the work table two or three feet from the tools and incubation slants. All dirt and slime is removed from the cap and its entire surface swabbed with 7% iodine solution. The cap is anchored by inserting three dissecting needles into its sides to form a flat tripod. An X-acto blade is steralized with an alcohol lamp flame, then allowed to cool. The outer skin is cut away from the cap. Small pieces of mushroom flesh are carved out and placed each one in its slant immediately. This is done by lightly spearring the piece with a sharply pointed triangular X-acto blade. The cap of the slant is lifted just enough to drop the piece onto the center of the lower 1/3 of the agar medium. The cap is then closed on slant immediately and returned to slant to 17° angle rack. Direct or shaded lighting is used depending upon the species. This is best

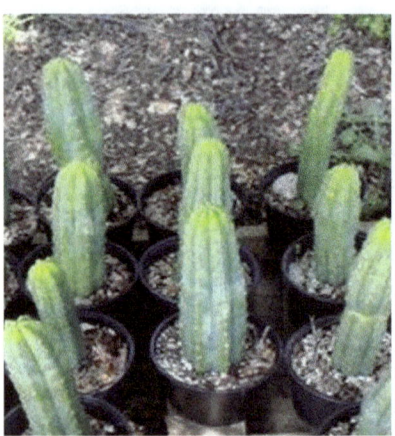

Growing mescaline cacti

determined by having taken note of the light or shade conditions under which it was found growing.

For accuracy in selecting the correct harvesting time for peak psilocybin production a home made incubating box is used. Wide spectrum GRO-LUX lamps are set for 12 hours on and 12 off. Thermostatic temperature control is set at 75° F. After a few days there will be a thread-like mass of white fibers—the mycelium—radiating out from the inoculum—the implanted piece of mushroom flesh. These fibers may later turn blue or bluish-green. Each slant is examined daily with a magnifying glass. If other fungus or bacterial cultures are observed, that slant is discarded. If the contaminating culture is not too near the psilocybe inoculum scooping it out with a sterilized platinum wire loop and putting a drop of 15 parts streptomycin/1 part aureomycin on the previously contaminated area may help. If the undesirable colony takes over again that slant is discarded.

One mushroom will provide many pieces of inoculum depending on the size and how is sliced. Setting up several slants is advised. When some fail others succeed. On the seventh day after inoculation the pH of a sample culture is tested. One with mycelial color and size is about typical of most of the others is selected. A small amount of the culture medium is withdrawn and smeared on the pH paper. The pH factor may have dropped toward greater acidity—as low as pH 3.7. This is a favorable sign of greater psilocybin production. Usually the maximum psilocybin content occurs between the seventh and the ninth days of cultivation. After that the pH factor rises sharply and the psilocybin content decreases rapidly. By the eleventh day, although the mycelium may grow a little more, the pH may be as high as 7.5 and the percentage of psilocybin may drop to less than half of what it was on the seventh day. If for some reason the mycelium can not be harvested immediately, its metabolism is suspended by putting the slants in the refrigerator.

Some warm water may be used to dissolve the agar in order to harvest the mycelium by filtering the medium through a flannel cloth. The mycelium is then dried in an oven at less than 200° F. The dried mycelium will contain about 1% psilocybin and/or psilocin and may be eaten as is or the alkaloids may be extracted with methanol. Upon harvesting a new batch is inoculated with pieces of mycelium from the previous batch. Then mushroom-hunting all over again is not necessary. The harvesting and re-inoculating can go on forever. In a small room one a thousand or more doses of psilocybin per week can be produced

GROWING PEYOTE AND OTHER PSYCHEDELIC CACTI

Peyote and San Pedro two contain mescaline. Peyote is illegal in some states, but there is at present no federal law prohibiting it. Constitutional law, however, has decided that the First Amendment's guarantee of religious freedom supersedes state laws of prohibition and that therefore members of the Native American Church—mostly Indians—may employ this sacrament in their religious rituals

San Pedro—*Trichocereus pachanoi*—contains mescaline, but because of the wording of the law it was still legal—at the time of this writing. Also its taste is not nearly as bitter as peyote, nor does it contain the same nauseating alkaloids.

Other cacti that contain mescaline, but are still legal, are: *Trichocereus terscheckii, T. Werdermannianus, and T. macrogonus.*

Other cacti containing alkaloids related to mescaline are *Cereus alacriportanus, C. forbesii, C. glaucus, C. peruvianus, C. peruvianus monstruosus, Echinopsis eyriesii, E. rhodotricha, Helianthocereus huascha, H. pasacana, H. poco, Trichocereus bridgesii, T. camaraguensis, T. candicans, T. lamprochiorus, T. peruvianus, T. schickendantzii, T. spachianus, Cereus jamacaru, Stetsonia coryne, Gymnocalycium gibbosum, and G. multiflorum.*

Cacti containing macromerine—about one-fifth the potency of mescaline are: *Coryphantha macromeris (Donana) and C. runyonii.*

The Huichols, Tarahumaras and other peyote-worshipping tribes of Mexico have at least 22 different species of cacti other than *Lophophora williamsii* which they also call peyote and employ as such. Among them are *Ariocarpus kotschoubeyanus, A. retusus*—also known as "tsuwiri," or "false peyote" are said to be more powerful than ordinary peyote and can be a bad trip, *4. fissuratus*—same as *Mammillaria fissurata*; locally called "sunami"; also said to be more powerful than peyote, *Mammillaria micromeris*—known as "mulato" and used for widening the eyes to see sorcerers, prolonging life and giving speed to runners), *Astrophytum asterias, A. capricorne, A. myriostigma,Aztekium ritterii, Dolichothele longimamma, Obregonia denegrii, Pelecyphora aselliformis, Solisia pectinata, Epitheliantha micromeris, and Pachycereus pecten-aboriginum (known as "cawe".*

GROWING CACTI FROM THE SEED

To grow cacti form seed a starting soil is prepared from one part dry dusty leaf mold and nine parts dry, gritty builder's sand. The leaf mold is sifted through a screen that has 22 to 24 holes per inch. Only that which passes through the screen is used. Sand is sifted through the same screen. Only sand that does not pass through the screen is used—i.e., the soil is made of fine leaf mold and coarse sand. The mixture is baked in the oven for one hour at 400 degrees to kill fungus, bacteria and weed seeds, then stored in a clean container while cooling.

Seed pans or flower pots between two and four inches diameter and no deeper than two inches are needed. If they have been previously used they are sterilize in the oven. The holes in the pots are covered with a small piece of cotton wool and a few strands of cotton are pulled through the hole to act as a wick. The cotton is gently pressed down on top but not packed too hard. Damp, unsifted sand—not the mixture— is sprinkled over the cotton to just cover it and pressed very gently.

Pots are filled with seeding mixture to 1/3 inch from the top without pressing. Instead pots are tapped on the table to level the soil. If soil is higher in the center a little soil is sprinkled around the edges. Most of the psyche-delic cacti have medium size seeds, which are scattered thinly over the surface of the soil. Then pots are stood in a baking tin half full of tepid water so the soil can soak up moisture in less than five minutes. Gritty sand is sprin-kled on the surface so that seeds are just covered. Pots are transferred to another baking tin that has about 1/16 inch of water on the bottom. This tin must be checked several times a day to see that the water remains at this level.

Peyote—*Lophophora*—and several other species have very small seeds—almost as fine as dust. These are sown by first sprinkling a thin layer of gritty sand over the surface of the soil. On top of this the seeds are scattered as thinly as possible. Most will fall between the sand grains. Pots are placed in a soak tray. After soil is moist-ened spray lightly with mist spray to help wash the seeds down among the grains, they are transferred to a germi-nating tray.

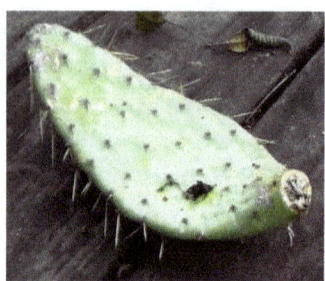

Cacti cutting

Some cacti have large, round seeds. These are sown individually with tweezers, placed about 1/4 inch apart with the germ eye down, pressed slighly into the soil with a dry finger, and covered with about 1/8 inch of gritty sand. Large flat seeds are handled similarly, but are planted vertically with the germ eye down.

If the humidity is not too high and if there is plenty of air circulation about the pots there should be no problem with damping off of the new seedlings. But if this is a problem a solution of 1/3 tsp. potassium hydroxyquinoline sulphate in one pint water may be used in the presoak tray. Cactus seeds are best planted between April and July. They germinate faster at this time and the young seedlings thrive better through the summer and early autumn when they don't have to contend with a cold winter draft.

A sheet of glass is placed over the pots while awaiting germination. Seeds may take from three days to three weeks to sprout and should not be exposed to direct sunlight. The temperature should be about 70° F. for most cacti. *Lophophora*—peyote—has difficulty sprouting if the temperature is too low, so between 80° and 90° F. is best.

After germination glass is removed and replaced by shade with muslin stretched over a frame. This frame is set parallel to the ground about six inches above the top of the pots to allow sufficient air flow. Young cactus seedlings are pale green to pink. If after two months from germination they are red or bronze they are getting too much light and need more shading with extra layers of muslin. If they become whitish or are elongated towards the light they are getting too much shade.

If pots are not absorbing enough water they should be soaked in deeper water just until top of soil becomes damp. Except for the first time when sowing small seeds the mist spray should not be used again until after three months and then it need only be used on warm, dry days. Tepid—never cold—water is always used with cacti. After from four to five months when the spines have formed on the seedlings the shading is removed for one or two hours each morning. Bottom watering is stopped and a watering can with a fine sprinkler is used twice a week—more in hot weather. Empty seed cases on the soil are removed so that they do rot and disease the plants.

When winter approaches the plants are moved indoors. They may be kept near a window during the day for sunlight and warmth, but are moved away from possible drafts before sundown. For most species the temperature should never drop below 40° F. Some thick-skinned species such as San Pedro, which grow high in the Andes, are fairly resistant to cold, but they do better if not subjected to this burden—especially during the seedling stage. Cacti require little water during the winter, but as seedlings it is best that they no be let to dry out or root damage can occur.

After the winter has passed the young plants can be pricked out by preparing transplant pots as follows: Cotton is stuffed into drain holes and covered with a thin layer of unsifted sand and about a 1/3 inch layer of leaf mold is placed on top. A tablespoon of bonemeal is evenly spread over the leaf mold and a teaspoon of crushed camphor sprinkled on top of it. Bonemeal gives slow, steady feeding and camphor repels harmful bugs. A mix of equal parts leaf mold and slightly coarse sand is prepared and baked in an oven as before. When cool it is spread on top of the camphor layer and filled to 1/2 inch from the top of the pot. The soil is leveled and smoothed by tapping, then 1/8 inch of coarse sand is sprinkled on the soil.

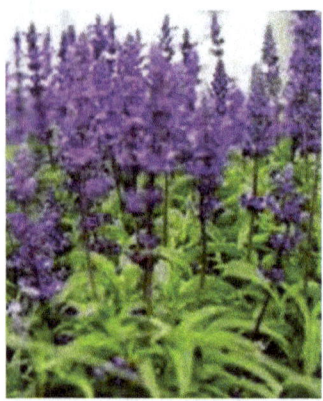

Salvia Divinorum

To prevent moss, the seedlings are watered the night before pricking out. Then on the following morning seedlings are removed by prying up gently with the back end of tweezers. Soil is left attached to roots. Tweezers are used to pick up plants at soil level and squeezed lightly. The new soil should be watered the night before to be a bit damp but not wet.

Holes are made in the new soil large enough to accommodate the roots and filled around each plant without pressing the soil down, which can disturb the roots. Later watering will settle the soil properly by using mist spray or watering can. Plants are placed one inch apart.Transplants are kept moist and shaded throughout the summer. Full light stops growth and turns plants bronze.

It is all right if the sand on top is dry most of the time as long as the soil is moist on the bottom. This can be checked by taking samples of leaf mold through the drain holes with tweezers.

The plants will grow rapidly during the spring and slowly through the summer. But the roots will be developing when the upper plants are not. In the autumn the plants will have another period of rapid growth.

After the second winter cacti can be transferred individually to larger pots or to their permanent location. A good soil mix for this is: 1 part loam, 1 part sand, 1 part leaf mold. To each gallon of this mix 4 heaping teaspoons of bonemeal, 3 of gypsum and 1 of superphosphate are added The two latter substances promote flowering, which is necessary to produce new seeds. Winter rest with minimum watering is also important for seed production. As before old and new locations are watered the night before transplanting.

GROWING CACTI FROM CUTTINGS

Growing cacti from seeds is a long process. After the first year most plants will be little more than 1/2 inch tall. More growth will be seen in the second year. Many prefer to grow cacti from cuttings rather than from seeds. To do this first allow cuttings to dry a few days in a dry, shady location.

The tender, exposed portion where the cut was made should dry to a corky texture before they are planted or else rotting may occur. A sterilized mix of 3 parts sand, 1 part leaf mold and 1 part loam is put in a pot with good

drainage. Then the pot is placed in a soak tray, allowing soil to become moist but not soggy. Before planting the bottom of the cutting may be dipped in a rooting mix such as RootOne.

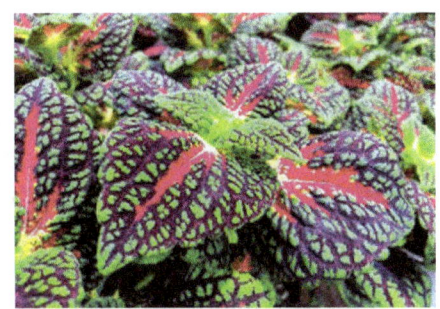

Coleus

RootOne contains hormones that promote root growth and fungicide to prevent rotting. The cutting is placed in the soil to a depth where the soil gives it adequate support. The soil should be kept slightly but evenly moist.

After several weeks or a month the plant will show signs of perking up and increased growth. This indicates that roots have formed. Water can be somewhat increased at this time. Plants should be kept away from hot sunlight until roots have formed. As plants grow offshoots will form. In the case of columnal cacti such as San Pedro some of these can be broken off when over five inches long and planted as cuttings. Side growths of low-growing cacti such as peyote and Donana can be separated and replanted.

TROUBLESHOOTING DISEASES AND DISORDERS

Plants should be inspected regularly for insects and other problems. Aphids and mealy bugs are fairly common especially on coryphanthas, rebutias and other soft-skinned cacti. These can be destroyed by brushing or spraying the entire plant with isopropyl rubbing alcohol. Scale insects which appear as brown, hard-shell spots about pinhead size can be scraped off with a toothpick if there are not too many.

Alcohol brushing is also effective. Red spiders usually occur only when conditions are dry. Sufficient humidity prevents their attacks. All of the above problems can be handled with nicotine sulfate, but this substance may be absorbed into the plant. The plants should be watered the day before spraying—including alcohol spraying and kept in the shade for several hours after spraying.

If plants become stunted and pale the roots should be checked. If rotted the roots are trimmed off and replanted in fresh soil. Such rotting may be due to overwatering or to microscopic nematode worms. If the plant is yellow it may be getting too much heat, or it may be suffering from an iron deficiency from over-alkaline soil. Soil pH should be tested. It should be a little on the acid side. If it is anywhere from neutral to alkaline, iron chelates should be added to soil.

Pale color on new growth may be due to root injury. If this is the case, damaged roots should be removed and repotted. If the plants become thin and elongated it may be the result of insufficient light.

Failure to bloom or the dropping of flower buds may be due to either inadequate winter rest, excessive cold, drafts or temperature fluctuation. Or it may be caused by too much nitrogen in the soil. If this is the problem low-nitrogen, high-phosphorus fertilizers can be added.

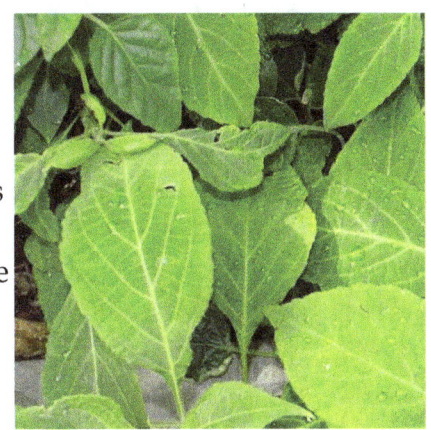

Salvia Divinorum

When harvesting cacti the root and some of the plant should be left intact so that it can grow anew. If dried for storage, it must be done immediately in the sun or in an oven at 100° to 150° F to avoid spoilage.

PIPIZINTZINTLI (SALVIA DIVINORUM) AND COLEUS

When psilocybe mushrooms are not in season the Mazatec Indians of north-eastern Oaxaca employ the leaves of Salvia divinorum and coleus as substitutes. Sixty or more large leaves are required for a trip, and although the effect is not as overwhelming as with the mushroom it is a definite hallucinogen often producing kaleidoscopic colors and three-dimensional images. These effects come on more quickly and are shorter-lasting than those of the mushroom. The leaves must be chewed very well or thoroughly mashed with water in a bowl or a blender.

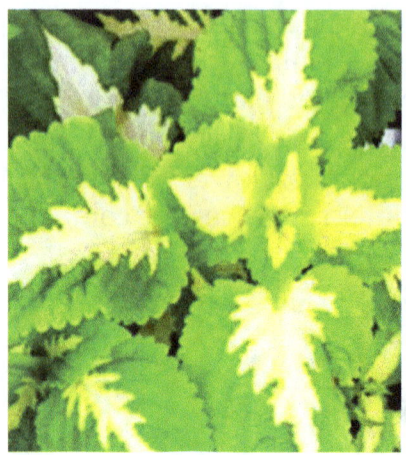

Coleus

Salvia is not in the habit of producing seeds and is always propagated vegetatively. The Indians usually grow their supply in remote ravines. The likelihood of obtaining *Salvia* shoots is very slender for most of us. But its close relatives *Coleus pumila* and *Coleus blumei* are readily available from nurseries and other stores as packaged seeds or full-grown potted house plants. Coleus can be raised from either the cutting or the seed.

Seeds are started indoors in a seed flat by scattering the seeds evenly on the surface and covering with 1/8 inch of fine soil. The flat must be kept well-watered but not soggy. Coleus sprouts best at about 75° F. The seeds usually germinate in about two weeks.

Some companies sell packages of coleus seeds in which the individual seeds are encased in a round gray clay-like substance about the size of a bee-bee. This supposedly makes planting easier and facilitates germination. I have tested these against normal, uncoated coleus seeds from the same company that were purchased the year before this innovation came out and found that the treated seeds took twice as long to sprout as the untreated kind. Also there were far fewer seeds in the treated pack than in the untreated one, although because of the bulky coating, the former appeared at first glance to contain more.

After all danger of frost has passed the plants can be transplanted outdoors in partial shade about 12 inches apart or potted individually and kept in a patio or as house plants. They must be watered regularly.

When plants are about six inches tall the upper half of

the stems are broken off and stuck into in a glass of water. After a week or two when roots appear on these plants are planted in soil. Meanwhile the plants from which the cuttings were removed will fork out into two more branches. This cutting and branching may be continued indefinitely on both the new plants and the new branches when these have attained the proper length. This gives many plants with abundant foliage.

Coleus plants are very beautiful and in a batch of mixed seeds one will hardly find any two that are exactly alike. Because of this it would be a shame to ravage an entire plant just to get high. Rooting of cuttings gives hundreds of copies of each original, and the destruction of a few plants will not seem so terrible. The Mazatecs used to employ the entire plant for divination, but now they use only the leaves. I have found the stems to be as active as the leaves and suspect that the reason for this new practice is conservational since fresh leaves grow where old ones have been removed.

When flower spikes appear they can be clipped off and used for tripping. If they are not removed they will sap the plants' energy. After this the plant may complete its life cycle and wither. Regularly clipped coleus plants can last forever. I collect the spikes along with fresh leaves that have fallen or broken off and keep them in a plastic bag in my freezer until there are enough for a trip.

The active components are preserved and the freezing and thawing causes the plant cells to rupture and collapse making the juices more accessible. These leaves and other pieces must be used immediately after removal from the freezer or they will quickly decompose.

Scientists have not identified the active substance in coleus and *S. divinorum*. Another plant of the same family—Labiatae or mint family—called *Lagochilus inebrians* is used as an intoxicant in Central Asia. A crystalline substance having the structure of a polyhydric alcohol has been isolated from the dried leaves of this little shrub. The yield was about 3%. The active material in coleus and *S. divinorum* appears to be unstable. I have tried both ingesting and smoking the dried leaves of coleus, but these had little or no effect.

Sometimes aphids will contaminate coleus plants. Ladybugs will usually keep the aphid population down. Ant traps can be placed in the vicinity of the plants because ants bring aphids. Intercropping with garlic and onions sometimes discourages aphids. If the plants become thoroughly overrun with these bugs it may be necessary to resort to more drastic methods, but chemical insecticides should not be used. One method is to submerge infested plants in a tub of water for about two hours. Aphids are slow to drown. This procedure can be repeated every four or five days for two weeks to destroy young aphids from eggs which remain on the plants after the previous dunking. Another method is to spray the plants with isopropyl rubbing alcohol. Get at the under-sides of the leaves is important, which is the aphid's favorite spot. After spraying the plants must dry off outside or in a well-ventilated place. They should not be exposed to direct sunlight immediately after spraying. Plants should be watered thoroughly right before spraying.

Coleus tends to grow more profusely when kept in a somewhat shallow pot. If the pot is too large the plant concentrates its energies on root growth rather than on foliage development. They seem to do better in pots than in gardens unless there is a layer of rock and gravel six or eight inches below the surface of the soil. The curtailed root development of a shallow-potted plant may eventually be insufficient to support the abundant foliage produced. Or the roots may become crowded. You will know if this is happening because the new leaves will be small and the color of the whole plant will take on a washed-out appearance. In this case plants eed to be repot in a larger container.

INCREASING THE LYSERGIC ACID CONTENT IN MORNING GLORIES AND HAWAIIAN BABY WOOD ROSE

The seeds of psychoactive varieties of Morning Glory and Hawaiian Baby Wood Roses are sometimes difficult to obtain. At one time you could purchase inexpensively a five-pound sack of these seeds; enough for hundreds of trips. Now, although there are no specific laws governing their sale, most of the seed companies have taken it upon themselves—usually with some pressure from local authorities—to pro-tect us from our freedom of choice by refusing to sellbulk quantities of these seeds. Some companies are pushing non-active variet-ies or treating active seeds with toxins which can make one deathly ill if consumed. There is clearly only one

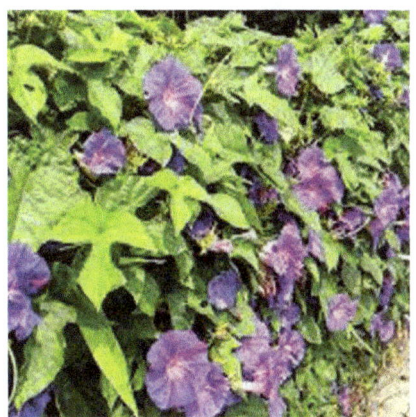

Common Morning Glory

immediate answer to these meddlesome acts of dictator-ship. People can grow their own. This is actually a happy solution to the problem for several good reasons:

1) Morning glories grow easily and profusely with very little care.

2) Not just the seeds, but the entire plant except for the roots contains psychoactive lysergic acid amides. These parts yield less on a weight-for- weight basis than the seeds, but because there is a larger portion of leaf and stems than seeds per plant there is a greater total yield per plant from the non-seed parts. It might be difficult to consume enough of these parts for a trip, but if one is

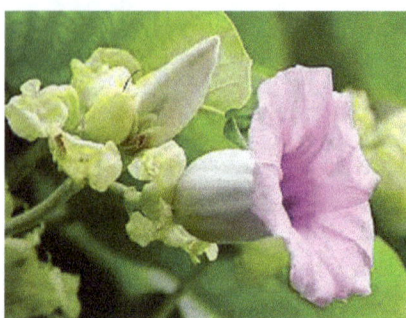

Hawaiian Baby Wood Rose

so inclined it would be worth the effort to extract alkaloids.

3) The proportion of these amides in the plant and seeds can be increased with certain growing techniques.

Remember: it is legal to grow morning glories. Small packs of the seeds are still available at some stores. But these seeds are becoming more and more scarce, so get them while you can. Brothers and sisters all over the country who do not want to submit to unconstitutional dictatorship can begin planting now.

Some of the harvested seeds may be used for tripping but some should be saved for next year's planting. The active varieties of morning glory and wood rose are in danger of becoming near extinct. In the name of God and Nature it is our duty as men and women to save the species.

When buying commercial packs of morning glory seeds avoid the following non-psychoactive varieties: Crimson Rambler, Sunrise Serenade, Rose Marie, Tinkerbell's Petticoat, Scarlett O'Hara, Candy Pink, Cornell, Royal Crown, Darling, Moon Vines, Cardinal Climber, Hearts and Honey, Cypress Vine, Mina Sanguinea.

If Latin names are given—see the reverse side of the pack—avoid: *Ipomoea purpurea, I. nil, I. alba, I. triloba, I. sloteri, I. quamoclit, I. coc-cinea, I. lindheimeri, I. muricata, I. turpethum, I. maxima, I. arborescans, Convolvulus tricolor, C. siculus, C. sepium.*

Use only Heavenly Blue, Pearly Gates, Flying Saucers, Wedding Bells, Summer Skies, Blue Star—all varieties of *Ipomoea violacea*, Badoh Negro, Ololiuqui, *Rivea corymbo-*

sa—Mexican morning glories. These last three are difficult to obtain in the United States.

Different environmental conditions produce seeds and plants with varying quantities of psychoactive alkaloids and amides. The likely range in any species may fall between .005% and .079% total indole alkaloids in different batches of seeds. Freshly harvested seeds are best. As the months pass stored seeds lose both their viability and their psychoactive properties. Broken or damaged seeds also swiftly lose both of these powers.

Seeds are sown in their permanent location after danger of frost is past. The seed has a hard protective coat and may be slow to germinate. To hasten germination seeds are soaked in water overnight. Some experts advise cutting or filing the side of the seed farthest from the germ eye just enough that some white appears. I have tested both methods and found that the soaked seeds sprout faster and have a better chance of survival than the scratched seeds.

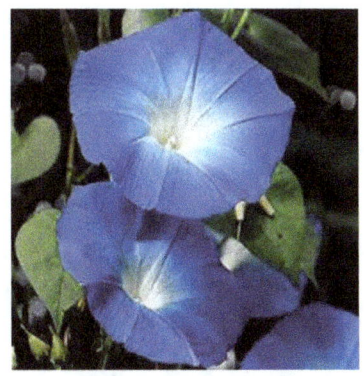

Morning Glory

Seeds are planted 1/2 inch deep under fine soil, not less than six inches apart. A fence, trellis or strings to support the fast-growing vines is needed. Stopping water for a few days if, at maturity, the vines do not seem inclined to produce flowers, may help. Generally cutting back on watering after that, but not so much that the plants wilt will hasten blooming. After that normal watering is resumed.

Morning glories grow easily with very little care. The challenge, however, is to get them to produce a maximum percentage of alkaloids. One factor influencing this is soil chemistry. Soil can be tested with a soil test kit, available

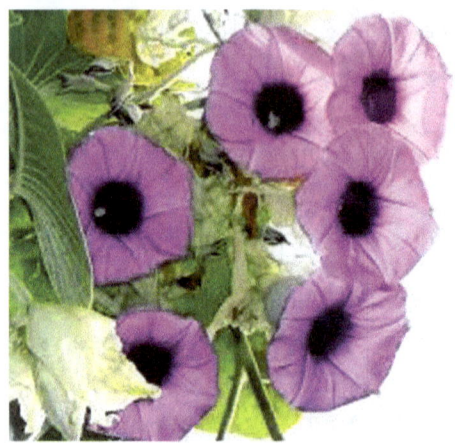

Hawaiian Baby Wood Rose

for a low price at most nurseries. The soil should have a pH factor of about 6.5, a high phosphate and low potassium content. High phosphate concentration increases indole alkaloid formation. Low potassium content of about 1.5 parts to 100 parts dry soil aids free tryptophan accumulation and biosynthesis. It also produces a low indoleacetic acid content, which means that more indole alkaloids will be formed. This is accomplished by using sodium nitrate instead of potassium nitrate for a nitrogen source and sodium hydrophosphate instead of potassium hydrophosphate to increase the phosphate content.

Experiments show that certain plant hormones have a positive influence on the alkaloid potency of morning glories. A solution of one gram gibberellic acid in one quart water can be used on the soil around the roots once every two weeks. This treatment is started while plant is in the seedling stage. Only a few drops are used at first and the amount is increased as the plant size increases so that when the plant is full size up to 1/2 ounce of solution per treatment.

Gibberellic acid stimulates growth as well as alkaloid production. It also delays maturity and inhibits flower and seed production. Therefore its use must be discontinued several weeks before flowering time. Further experiments indicate that growth-inhibiting auxins such as alpha naphthalene acetic acid can also increase the alkaloidal yield. There is a need for much study of the effects of different combinations of these substances on the potency of morning glory seeds. We are interested in hearing the results of experiments. But even without the use of hormones and auxins amazing results can be achieved by employing the soil chemistry control method described herein.

There are some species of plants which have mutually beneficial influences on other species that are intercropped or planted nearby. Morning glories prosper well when intercropped with corn, soybeans, or sorghum.

The Hawaiian Baby Wood Rose—*Argyreia nervosa*, which belongs to the same family as the morning glory, may contain from three to six times as much lysergic acid amides as its cousins. It can be grown as easily as morning glories and its alkaloid production is influenced by the same conditions. Planting instructions given for morning glories should be followed, but bear in mind that these are tropical plants and do not favor chilly climate. They will do fine during warm summers or in a heated greenhouse. The seeds should be as fresh as possible because older seeds tend to lose their viability.

After opening a pod—four seeds to the pod—only the largest and firmest seeds are selected for planting The others are fine for tripping. Wood rose seeds are more susceptible to bacterial decay than are morning glories. It is best the soil and germinating water is steralized beforehand.

The larger wood rose does not contain as much psychoactive alkaloids as the baby wood rose. Also its pods are more difficult to crack open. But in lieu of the smaller variety it may be used. Both kinds are available at some flower shops.

It can be difficult for an amateur to discern the different species, and some mushrooms, which almost look like the kind you may be seeking can be quite deadly. Some people have smuggled spores from Mexico and South America. This is not hard to do since they are fine as dust.

PART THREE:
Herbal Aphrodisiacs

What is an aphrodisiac? Everybody talks about aphrodisiacs, but no one seems to know anything about them. Many so called "experts" insist that there is no such thing as an aphrodisiac. It is not surprising that only a few decades ago many of the same "experts" assured us that the idea of sexual pleasure and orgasm in the female was "totally absurd". Our own definition of aphrodisiac includes substances which do any one or several of the following things.

Produce erections in the male, arouse sexual feeling by stimulation of the genitals or nervous system, increase sensual awareness, relax inhibitions, augment physical energy, strengthen the gonads or other glands involved in sex, improve sexual health, increase the production of semen, help conquer impotence and frigidity—bearing in mind that these maladies are frequently of psychological-origin, overcome sexual exhaustion, and prevent premature ejaculation. This book is about the chemistry of sex, and natural substances that influence it.

We will explore not only aphrodisiac materials as defined above, but also tonics which aleviate female complaints, ease childbirth and add years to your sex life. We have also included a comprehensive chapter on nutrition and sex and disclosed for the first time a revolutionary method of birth control.

UNDESIRABLE APHRODISIACS

Since cantharides—Spanish Fly—is the most famous aphrodisiac in human conversation let us deal with it first. It is the pulverized wing parts of a species of beetle *Lytta vesicatoria*. If taken internally even in minute doses it causes extreme irritation of the genitals, fever, painful urination and possible bloody discharge. Sometimes—but not often —it produces an illusion of insatiable sexual desire. WARNING! Spanish Fly is unreliable, dangerous, often fatal, and nearly always causes permanent or long term injury.

L-DOPA, (-)-3-(3,4-dihydroxyphenyl)-L-alanine, a new drug for the treatment of Parkinson's Disease increases sexual desire in some individuals. It is an unreliable aphrodisiac with many unfavorable side effects too numerous to list here.

In 1970 workers piping a new kind of gas into homes in Harrogate, England noted that it made them feel drunk and increased sexual desire. Little else is known about this gas as yet.

PCPA, *p-chlorophenylalanine*, causes hypersexual aggression in laboratory animals, but it also makes them vicious and can have harmful effects on several body organs. Dr. Nicolas Venette, a 17th century medical author proclaimed borax, sodium tetraborate an excellent aphrodisiac. I do not advise experimentation with this corrosive chemical.

Amyl nitrite ampules, known as "poppers" were originally intended as a heart stimulant for people with cardiac disorders. They are now popular among "sexy" people. An ampule is broken open and sniffed at the point of orgasm. It gives a brief flash for about 30 seconds that intensifies sexual climax. They are relatively harmless if used occasionally, but I suggest that you not get hung up on them or any chemical stimulants.

YOHIMBE

(*Corynanthe yohimbe*)

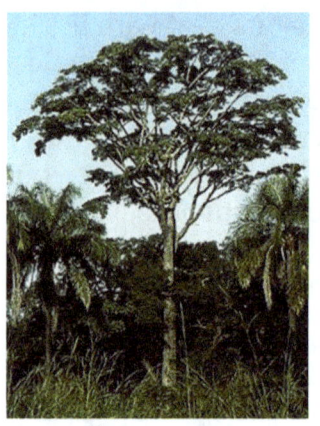

Yohimbe Tree

Earlier in Herbal Highs, I spoke of Yohimbe and its psychedelic effects. I briefly mentioned que-brachine, an aphrodisiac drug derived from the bark of this West African tree by reacting yohim-biline, one of its alkaloids, with hydrochloric acid. In effect this is a way of shortcutting the diges-tion and assimilation of the alka-loid. When you drink the tea the alkaloids, yohimbine and yohim-biline must react with the hy-drochloric acid in your digestive juices so that they become soluble and can be assimilated into your body.

Recently at Stone Kingdom, we made a wonderful discovery: If you add 1000 mg of ascorbic acid—vitamin C—to each cup of Yohimbe bark tea, the two will react to produce yohimbine and yohimbiline ascorbate, a very soluble and assimilable form of the two alkaloids. By doing this you have a smoother and better trip with no tendency towards the slight nausea which sometimes accompanies the use of the tea. It comes on quicker too—10-15 minutes instead of 30~45. Also its aphrodisiac qualities are more pronounced. Yohimbe brings blood to the pelvic area and by stimulating the spinal nerves, encourages erections in the male as well as heightening sensual pleasure for both sexes. It acts as a stimulant to the parasympathetic nervous system in a way that brings

There is nothing in the influence of any aphrodisiac that lovers cannot eventually learn to do by themselves.

out profound emotional feelings. During sex, lovers feel as though their bodies were disolving and merging into One another.

Orgasm under the influence of yohimbe is beyond belief. Its effect is so powerful that men and women who suffer from psychological impotence and frigidity usually overcome their mental and physical barriers and experience a really great climax. A word to the wise, however: yohimbe is meant to be used for pleasure on occasion or, in cases of impotence and frigidity, until natural confidence is restored. Remember: There is nothing in the influence of any aphrodisiac that lovers cannot eventually learn to do by themselves.

A man and woman who turn on to each other is the world's most powerful aphrodisiac.Yohimbe, like any other aphrodisiac is pleasurable and enlightening. It can teach things about your body and its capacities that you may never have suspected and may help to free you from use of the physically manifested inhibitions that we have inherited from the enormous superego of past generations. But don't let it or anything else become a crutch, for this would not be freedom, but only another form of slavery.

YOHIMBE TEA

Simmer 5-8 tsp. of shaved bark or 3-6 tsp. of powdered bark for 5 minutes in 1 pint of boiling water. Strain or filter, then add Vitamin C. Earlier in Herbal Highs, 6-10 tsp. were recommended, but with the vitamin less is required. Yohimbe sometimes produces tingly feeling in the genitals and pleasurable warm shivers through

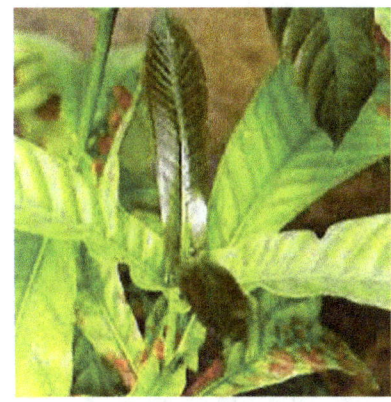

Yohimbe Leaves

the back during intercourse. It is not physically addicting and there are no known harmful side effects. However, it should never be taken with alcohol because this combination is toxic.

DITA
(Alstonia scholaris)

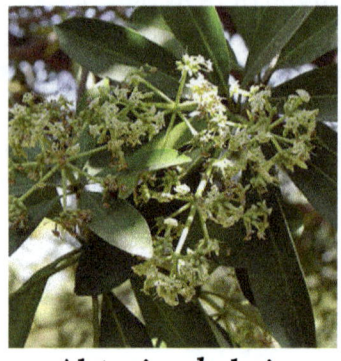

This tree of the Apocynaceae—dogbane—family comes from Eastern Asia and the Philippines. It has attractive white, funnel shaped flowers and is rarely seen in America. The bark used as a tea has long been a standard and effective folk medicine in Asia for lessening the distress of women's monthlies.

Alstonia scholaris

In India a tonic is made from the seeds and bark. The seeds—but not the bark—are a strong aphrodisiac. They contain a powerful alkaloid, chlorogenine, $C_{21}H_{20}N_2O_4$, that helps a man retain erection and delay orgasm during intercourse. The seeds are crushed in water and soaked overnight.

NIGHT BLOOMING CEREUS

(Cereus grandiflorus, Mill)

This fragrant flowered cactus can be found in Mexico, Jamaica, and the American South West. Although it is often sold under the name "cactus flowers". It is the stem that contains the active ingredient, a drug with heart stimulating properites similar to digitalis. It is noncumulative, however. It has been used in the treatment of prostrate diseases, nervous menstrual headache, and to overcome sexual exhaustion. For the latter about 1/2 gram of the fresh plant is chewed or crushed in 2 cc. of brandy and allowed to soak for a few minutes before drinking. The active component is alcohol soluble. Although the fresh plant is best, in Jamaica it is usually sold crushed and preserved in alcohol. In the American Southwest the Indians prefer to use the root.

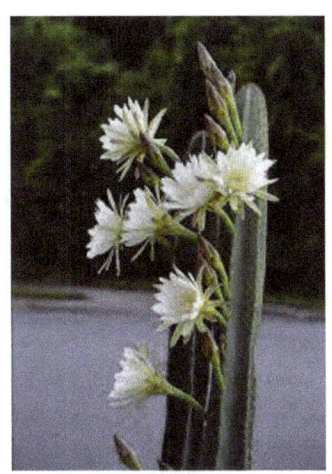

Night Blooming Cereus

I don't know if there is any similarity, but the Indians of Bolivia concoct an elixer from a local thornless cactus that is said to keep a man young up until the time of his death.

SENSITIVE PLANT

(Ikimosa pudica)

This shrub—also known as humble plant or touch-me-not—is found in Mexico, Central America and Brazil. It is sometimes cultivated in the United States as an indoor and greenhouse curiosity.

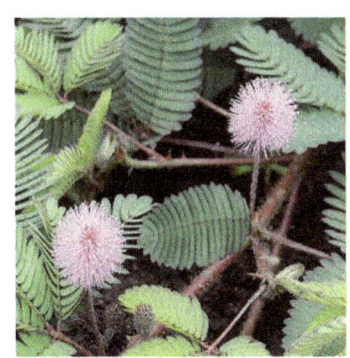

Sensitive Plant

The leaves of this plant are arranged in a sort of herringbone pattern along the leaf stem. If touched lightly they immediately fold together. The natives of the Amazon saturate the leaves with the root juices and plaster them to the soles of their feet or over their breasts to give them extended sexual power orgasm after orgasm. This may sound peculiar to our way of thinking, but there are a surprizing number of similar techniques employed in folk medicine through-out the world.

In India, for example, powdered henna is rubbed on the fingertips, scull and soles for one or two weeks as a cure for impotence and premature ejaculation. The fingertips are an excellent point of absorbtion as anyone who has handled large quantities of LSD well knows.

SARSAPARILLA

(Smilax officianalis)

For many centuries the Indians of Mexico have used an infusion from the roots of this tropical American vine as a cure for physical debility, weakness and impotence. White men generally regarded this treatment as a humorous example of superstitious medicine. Then in 1939, Dr. Emerick Solmo, a Budapest scientist living in Mexico discovered that the root was very rich in testosterone, the male sex hormone. Today most of the testosterone manufactured for pharmaceutical use is derived from sarsaparilla.

Medical testosterone comes in two forms: testosterone propianate, which is administered by injection; and methyl testosterone, which is given sublingually, that is the tablet is held under the tongue for a few minutes until it disolves and is absorbed into the buccal mucous lining of the mouth. It is not swallowed because the chemistry of the digestive fluids would interfere with the proper assimilation of the hormone. Testosterone is employed to bring on secondary male sex characteristics in cases of retarded adolescence and to enlarge an underdeveloped penis.

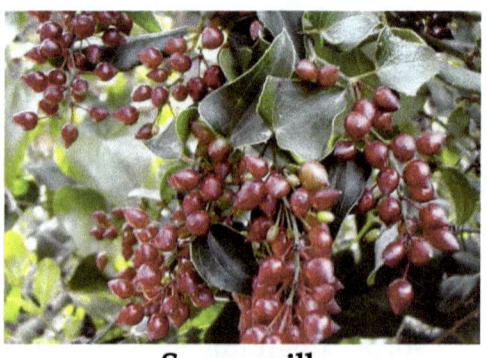

Sarsaparilla

For older men it is used to rejuvenate sex drive, over-come impotence and improve general health and energy. Some physicians have to a certain extent conquered baldness by rubbing testosterone on the scalp regularly for several months to a year. I have not had the time or opportunity to test the effects of sarsaparilla extractions on baldness, but it would be an interesting and harmless experiment for anyone who wished to try it.

If a man finds his sexual desires waning for physical —not psychological—reasons, the daily use of testoster-one will, in a matter of weeks not only restore his erotic interests, but also improve his general health, vigor, ap-pearance, muscle tone and productive energy. Curiously, however, if a man is already highly sexed the use of tes-tosterone while it improves health, muscle tone, etc. and greatly increases creative energy, it will slightly decrease his sexual desires—not enough to be regarded as impo-tence but enough to be noticeable.

Sarsaparilla also contains several other hormones including progesterone and cortin, an adrenal hormone that helps us to resist infectous disease and nervous depression.

SARSAPARILLA TEA

One or two heaping tablespoons of the dried root is sim-mered in a pint of water for five minutes. It will tend to foam up so be careful that it does not boil over. Strain the liquid and, bearing in mind what was said about the in-compatability of testosterone and the digestive acids. Take small sips and let them linger in the mouth for a minute before swallowing.

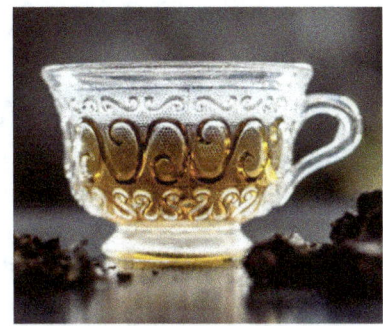

Sarsaparilla Tea

OPIUM

(Papaver somniferum)

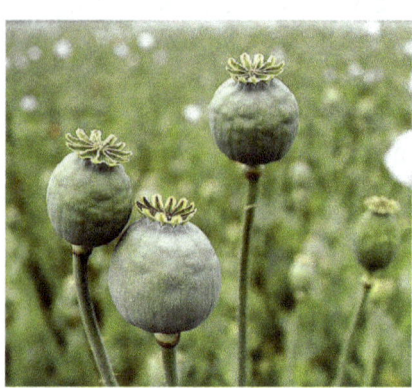

Opium

If used correctly opium can be a most excellent aphrodisiac. In moderate doses it opens one to erotic suggestions. All opium alkaloids have a stimulating influence on the spinal cord like that of strychnine, yohimbe and burra gokeroo in that they tend to produce erections. In addition the drug acts as both a stimulant and relaxant and excites voluptuous fantasies.

It has an anesthetizing effect on the penile nerves in the glans; not enough to deprive a man of sensual'pleasure but enough to delay orgasm. In the female, it anesthetizes the rectal and vaginal nerves and has often been used to make anal intercourse easier.

The simplest and least wasteful way to smoke opium is to place a tiny bead of it in the bowl of a long stemmed brass pipe. The bowl is held over a candle flame or alcohol lamp so that the flame barely licks over the top of the bowl. While tilting the stem at a 45 degree angle the lover inhales deeply and leisurely. Opium swells and bubbles when heated. In its melted state it tends to clog the pipe, but if the bead is not too large and the pipe is kept tilted this problem is lessened.

Although moderate doses are an effective aphrodisiac when given occasional use, more than just a few pipefuls has a reverse effect and weakens the libido. Excessive longterm use can be dangerous and debilitating and may destroy the sex drive. Constant and heavy use can become a habit difficult to break. And opium is illegal to possess.

GINSENG

(Panax schinseng)

For over 5000 years Oriental men have consumed ginseng root, daily to retain their virility. Many have been known to father children while in their seventies. *The Atherva Veda*—the ancient medical manual of India—says that it bestows on men both young and old the power of a bull.

It is, however, not merely a temporary genital stimulant. It is a rejuvenator and reactivator of not only the gonads but of all the endocrines and the entire organism. Soviet scientists have isolated from the root three major components: panaxin, panaquilom and schingenin, which in combination strengthens the heart and nervous system and increases the flow of hormones. The Russian scientists claim that the root gives off minute amounts of a unique type of ultra-violet radiation that stimulates the healthy growth of tissue especially in the endocrine system, and has a general healing and rejuvenating influence on the body. They call this subtle radioactive quality *mitogenic radiation*. Originally the plant was harvested from its natural habitat, but now that its agricultural peculiarities have been mastered it is mostly cultivated.

Importers have conspired to keep its cost far above what it should be. The highest quality, Imperial Ginseng, is available to only the wealthiest and most important Chinese. The next grade is Korean Ginseng. After that comes American Ginseng—a different species—*Panax quinquefolium*— that is sold mostly to Americans and poor Chinese. The lowest quality is Japanese Ginseng. Unfortunately many farmers have been sold Japanese seeds for Korean so the ginseng market has

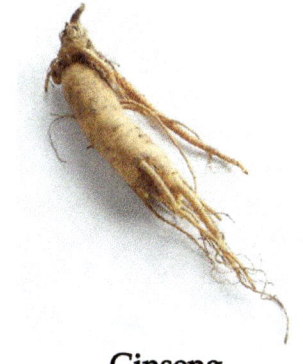

Ginseng

been badly adulterated. Ginseng grows slower wild than cultivated. Wild ginseng is usually not worth harvesting if it is less than ten years old. Three or four year old cultivated roots, however, will often outweigh 30 to 40 year old wild ones. Age increases quality and price.

The best way to use ginseng is to thoroughly chew a pinch every 3 or 4 hours. Saliva helps to activate its qualities. Some people like to make a tea from it by boiling 1 teaspoon of the root filaments in a pint of water for ten minutes. This is all right, but don't waste the pulp. It can be used over several times and after that it can be chewed and swallowed. Better than that if you can get the powdered root then mix 1/4 to 1/2 teaspoon in a cup of hot water.

Ginseng tea should be sipped slowly allowing small quantities of the liquid to linger in the mouth and mingle with the salivary fluids before swallowing. Its rejuvenating influence on older men is gradual over a period of months. I have observed that when younger men take ginseng its aphrodisiac effects are noticeable more immediately. It is equally beneficial to both sexes, but since Asia has always been a male oriented society more has usually been said of its value to that gender.

KOLA

(Cola nitida)

The natives of Sierra Leone and North Ashanti use the nut of this African tree as a nerve stimulant and aphro-

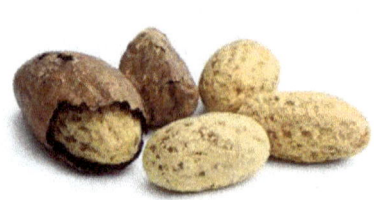

disiac. They either chew or grind and brew them as a beverage. The nut contains as much caffeine as coffee, but the kola oil is also a stimulant and regulator of metabolism,

Kola

A convenient and economical way to use kola is to put 1 teaspoon of powdered Kola and 2 teaspoons of honey in a cup and stir them into a paste. Then fill the cup with hot water, stir once more and sip slowly. Prepared this way it is a delicious beverage. Excessive use of coffee can weaken the sexual drive. Kola seems to lack many of the harmful properties of coffee, but it does contain caffeine so I do not advise indulging in more than one or two cups a day.

SAW PALMETTO

(Serenoa repens)

This stemless palm grows most commonly in south eastern North America, especially in Florida, where many people enjoy eating the fresh berries. The dried berries are excellent, too. They are very nutritious and act as a tonic for the glandular tissues. Saw Palmetto berries build strength and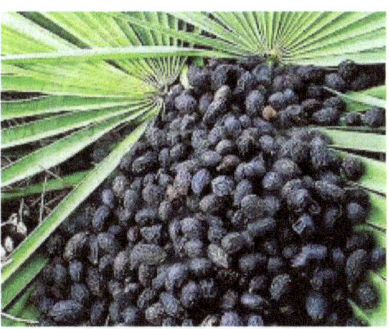

Saw Palmetto

healthy body tissue very rapidly and tend to normalize body weight. They are excellent for regaining health after any wasting illness and have an anticatarrhal influence on sore urinary passages. They are frequently used in cases of atrophy of the testes and mammary glands.

Some modestly developed young ladies claim to have noticed an increase in breast size after including the berries in their diet for a few months. However, they are most famous for their ability to increase the production of sperm in the male when taken regularly. In this sense saw palmetto can be regarded as a truly beneficial aphrodisiac.

At least a teaspoonful of berries should be eaten daily. They are most effective when taken along with damiana tea.

DAMIANA

(Turnera diffusa)

This plant is found in tropical America and Africa. It was discussed in Herbal Highs because smoking the leaves at the same time as drinking the tea produces a "grass like" high. The tea has definite aphrodisiac effects and is an excellent tonic for the reproductive organs of both sexes.

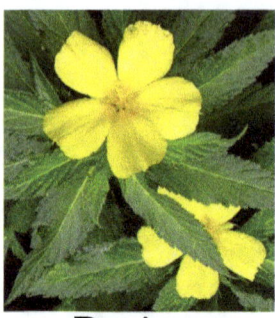

Damiana

Many women find that a cup of damiana tea taken an hour or two before intercourse helps them to get really immersed in the sex act-Both men and women have reported that a cup of the tea with a little honey taken before retiring tends to encourage amorous dreams. It makes a delightfully aromatic beverage that can be used regularly in place of tea or coffee without any harmful effects. In fact it is very healthful because of its tonic influence upon the genitals and nervous system.

Damiana is usually most effective used in combination with saw palmetto. One or two heaping tablespoons should be steeped for five minutes in a pint of water.

STRYCHNINE

(Strychnos nux vomica)

This tree grows in China, Burma, India and Australia. If used correctly in the proper dosage, strychnine, the alkaloid found in the seeds is an excellent medicine.It is useful as a stimulant and general tonic especially in combination with other materials. It has served as a remedy for neuralgia, diapepsia, debility, chronic constipation and impotence.

Its action in the latter case is effected by stimulation of the circulation, muscular system, and the spinal nerves. I can not, however, recommend it for use by unskilled hands. There is a very narrow margin between the useful and toxic dosages and tolerance varies considerably from one person to another. Because the percentage of the alkaloid within the seed can vary widely from tree to tree

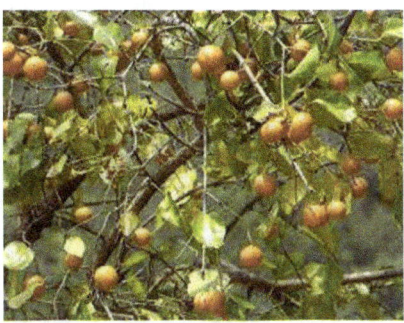

Strychnine

I will suggest no dosages for the raw material. There are other substances such as Yohimbe and Burra gokeroo that have action similar to strychnine but lack its dangers.

BURRA GOKEROO

(Pedalium murex)

In India the seeds of this plant are crushed and made into a tonic for the treatment of impotence. It also seems to have a beneficial effect on the genito-urinary passages especially in cases of mild infection and irritation. Some Asian doctors have used it successfully on older people who have difficulty containing their urine.

One part seeds are crushed and soaked for 24 hours in 20 parts water. The liquid is strained and and put up in bottles. One teaspoon is taken three times a day. It is best to keep the bottle refrigerated to prevent the tonic from spoiling. Or else add 1 part pure grain alcohol to 9 parts tonic. Burra gokeroo appears to have a strychnine like effect on the spinal cord which encourages erections, but apparently does not have the toxic dangers of the latter.

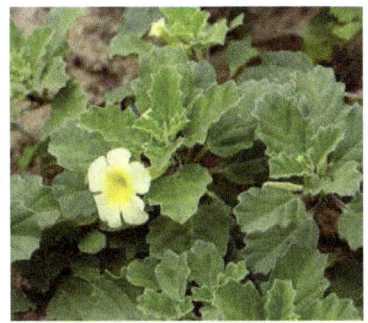

Pedalium murex

KELP

(Macrocystis pyrifera)

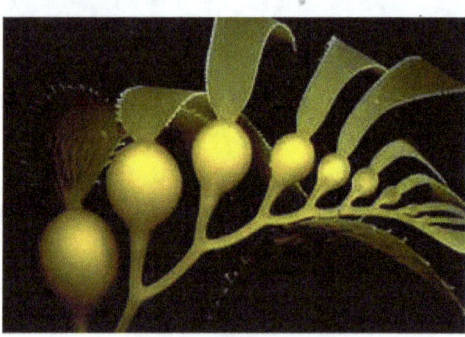

Kelp Seaweed

Kelp is a seaweed found in the waters along the California coast. It is rich in organic minerals essential to general glandular health, and contains ten times as much iodine as iodized salt. Iodine is essential to the healthy functioning of the thyroid gland. This gland produces a hormone needed to turn food into energy. Insufficient iodine can cause chronic fatique, mental sluggishness, irregular and profuse menstruation and decrease of libido or sex drive. One teaspoon of kelp daily will correct most deficiency induced thyroid abnormalities. Other substances needed for healthy thyroid functioning are protein, vitamins C, E and B complex.

A marvelous thyroid tonic can be made my mixing 1 teaspoon powdered kelp, 1 teaspoon wheat germ oil, 1 tablespoon yeast—from a health food store and 500 mg. vitamin C in a glass of tomato juice. Shake or stir well before drinking. Kelp has cumulative benefits. People who use it regularly soon notice a marked increase in both sexual and general energy. Another highly nutritive seaweed food is Dulse—*Halymenia edulis & H. palmata*. It is found along the British coast, and is one of the most well balanced mineral foods in the world. It can be used along with or instead of kelp.

RED CAPSICUM

(Capsicum frutescens)

This hot spicy red pepper is grown in India, Japan, Africa, the East Indies and tropical America. There are several qualities and potencies available. The most common is known in the markets as cayenne. It is regarded as one of the purest and most positive stimulants in herbal medicine.

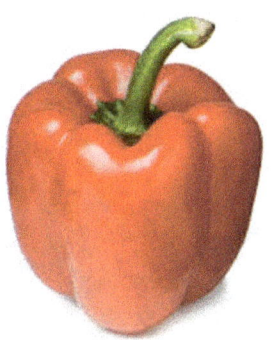

Red Capsicum

It helps to purify the system, increases and equalizes the blood circulation, produces natural body heat, and wards off colds. When used on food, it produces a strong burning sensation in the mouth but it does not cause any physical injury. Those who have not acquired a taste for it may prefer to put it into gelatin capsules. 30 to 125 mg. is the usual recommended dosage. Some people like to make a powerful stimulant blend of equal parts powdered Korean ginseng, ginger and capsicum. The daily use of capsicum or the blend quickly stirs up erotic energies.

COTTON ROOT

(Gossypium herbaceum)

The root bark of this herb from Asia Minor has been used for many centuries to encourage contractions in childbirth, ease labor pains and to bring on delayed monthlies. For this latter purpose it is safer and more effective than ergot. It is also useful for overcoming sex-

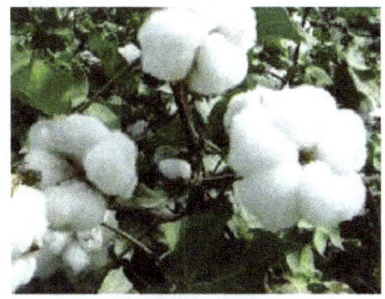

Cotton Plant

ual lassitude in either sex. Two ounces of the root bark
are added to one pint of boiling water for three minutes.
Strain the liquid and give doses of one wine- glassful no
more often than three hours apart.

FO-TI-TIENG

(Ilydrocotyle Aaiatica minor)

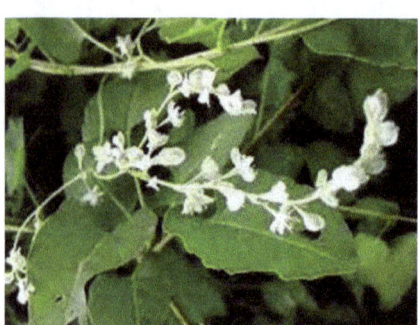

Fo-Ti-Tieng

The noted Chinese herbal-
ist Li Chung Yun, was full
of good advise on how to
retain ones youth, health
and sexual vigor through-
out life and live to a vital-
ly ripe old age. He advo-
cated strict vegetarianism,
believed that with the
exception of ginseng one
should eat only food that
grew above the ground
and recommended that one should keep a quiet heart, sit
calmly like a tortoise, walk sprightly like a pigeon, and
sleep soundly like a dog. But his most important prescription was the daily use of Fo-ti-tieng, a low growing plant
of the pennywort family found in the jungle marshes of
the Asian tropics.

Unfortunately this worthy gentleman died in 1933.
But I suppose we should not feel too badly because it is a
matter of record with the Chinese government that he was
born in 1677. Li was 256 at the time of his death and had
only recently married his twenty-fourth wife. He had his
own teeth and hair and looked about 50 when over 200.

Typically, the bulk of the scientific world preferred to
ignore someone like Li surpassed their understanding.
But there were exceptions: The well known French bio-
chemist, Jules Lepine found in the leaves and seeds of

this plant an alkaloid which has a rejuvenating influence on the nerves, brain cells and endocrine glands. Professor Menier of the Academis Scientifique near Paris made similar observations. The famous Indian sage and guru, Nanddo Narian at the age of 107 informed his followers that this herb contains a missing ingredient in man's diet without which we can never completely control disease and decay.

Short term experiments with Fo-ti-tieng, which in Chinese means elixer of long life, show that the daily use of 1/2 teaspoon of the powdered herb in a cup of hot—not boiling—water softens many signs of aging, such as lines and wrinkles, improves digestion and general health, and has a calming effect on the nerves while tremendously increasing physical and mental energies. Larger doses—1 or 2 tablespoons—act as an aphrodisiac with cumulative effects especially when sexual vitality is lagging.

MARIJUANA

(Cannabis indica)

Anything that generally turns you on to life is bound to turn you on to sexual pleasures. I think we all agree that sex and life are one. The aphrodisiac nature of marijuana has been recognized for many centuries. In India aphrodisiac bon-bons are made from the seeds and leaves of cannabis mixed with musk and honey. It is not that marijuana has any particular stimulating effect on the gonads, but rather that it relaxes the mind and body, diminishes unnecessary inhibitions, and opens one to sensual awareness. Recent scientific studies

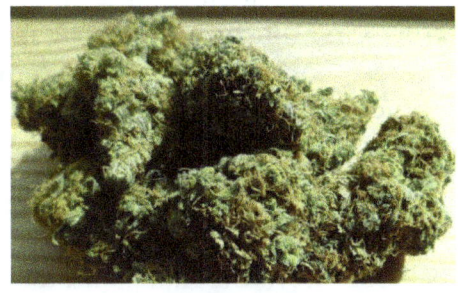

Marijuana

show that pot smokers engage in 60 to 80% more sexual activity than non-users.

There is a possible reverse effect, however, that should be mentioned: Marijuana and other psychedelics have a way of bringing out the truth. If a person is with someone merely because of general unspecific horniness, fear of loneliness or any other dishonest motivation rather than love or genuine sexual attraction, marijuana can turn one off instead of on because it makes one aware of the deception.

The two-sided effects of the more powerful psychedelics are even more pronounced. This does not mean that if your mate is tripping on grass or acid, but does not feel in the mood for love that you should necessarily assume that it is all over between the two of you. Psychedelics can sometimes turn a person inward to private contemplations. Often they bring on floods of creative thought that temporarily override all else. Generally, however, many couples find that a shared joint or a few tokes of hashish before bed time is a wonderful prelude to an evening of love.

OTHER APHRODISIAC HERBS

Wise men of ancient times including Aristotle, who held much influence with Alexander the Great, forbade the use of wild mint—*Mentha sativa*—by soldiers in times of war because it aroused them erotically and took away their animosity and courage to fight. In ancient Greece and Macedonia mint tea was made stronger than it is in our country.

The correct way to make mint tea as was done in Aristotle's day is to bring the water to boiling then remove the kettle from the flame and let it stand for one minute before pouring one pint of water over one ounce of the leaves. Let the leaves steep for three minutes with the lid on the teapot before serving. Never boil mint tea because that will evaporate the essence.

LIQUORICE ROOT

Ancient Egyptians, Hindus and Chinese were fond of liquorice root. The pharaohs enjoyed a vitalizing and refreshing beverage made of it called mai sus. The Chinese chewed the root to give them strength and endurance. The Hindus made a tea of it with milk and honey to increase their sexual vigor. The extracted juices of the fresh root

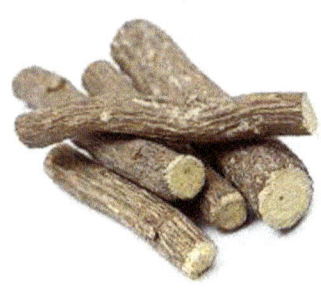

Liquorice Root

are best for this purpose. If this is not available a pound of the dried root can be cut into small pieces and boiled in 3 pints of water. Strain the liquid and boil down to one quart. Serve with honey and milk. This combination has been also found to be soothing for ulcers. In 1950 it was discovered that liquorice root contained substantial quantities of estrogen, the female sex hormone.

VANILLA BEAN ORCHID

Vanilla is another well known flavoring substance which has unquestionable aphrodisiac qualities. Madamme DuBarry used to serve it to her lovers to keep them perpetually ready. Obviously the small amounts of vanilla used to flavor ice cream and des-

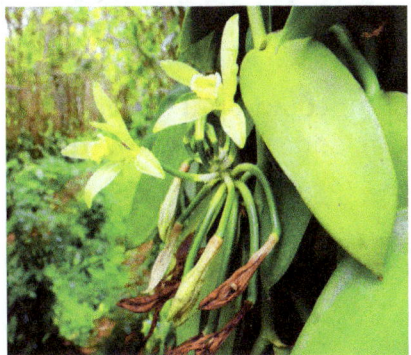

Vanilla Bean Orchid

serts are hardly enough to lead a person to the bedroom. Larger quantities are needed. If anyone wishes to experiment with this substance it is best that they begin with one or two pods and gradually increase the dose because excessive amounts of vanilla can have toxic effects. Vanilla flavoring is extracted from the bean pods of the vine, *Vanilla planifolia*, a member of the orchid family. Workers who handle these pods daily often develop severe skin irritation. It is curious that many scholars believe that Satyrion, the legendary aphrodisiac of the Greeks, was actually the root of orchishircina—another member of the orchid family—served in goats milk.

PIPER ANGUSTIFOLIUM

(Piper angustifolium)

Several plants of the pepper family have a history as aph-

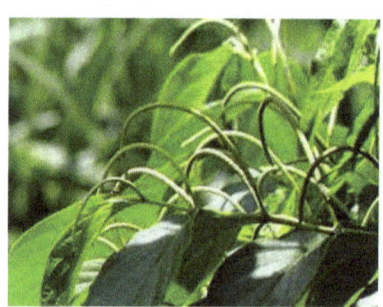

Pepper angustifolium

rodisiacs: Matico leaves—*Piper angustifolium*—have been used as a sex stimulant by the Peruvian Indians for many centuries. One talbespoon of leaves is added to each cup of boiling water. After a minute the pot is taken off the flame. It is then allowed to stand for half an hour. Then the liquid is strained and put outside in the cold air (a refrigerator will do), and later it is served chilled.

CUBEB PEPPER BERRIES

(Piper cubeba)

Cubeb pepper berries are well known for their ability to arouse libido. The dried berries can be run through a pepper grinder and used as a condiment or crushed and brewed as a tea. The stimulating component appears to be the volatile oil. This can be extracted with brandy or pure grain spirits.

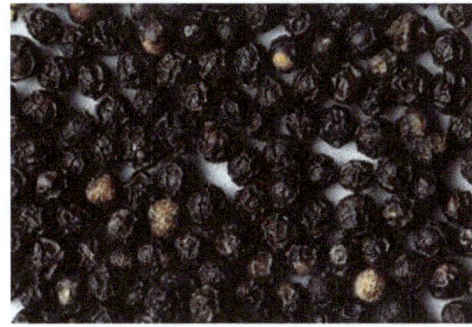

Cubeb Pepper Berries

In China an infusion of the leaves is used for exciting and strengthening the male organ. Another member of the pepper family is Kava-kava—*Piper mpfhvsfi. num*— described earlier in Herbal Highs seciton. The root of Kava-Kava is brewed as a pleasant and harmless narcotic beverage in the South Sea Islands. Alcohol extracts Kava resin and can be evaporated off. Saliva activates the resin. A dab during oral love makes a woman's clitoris feel warm and tingly.

SATOVARI

A juice extracted from the root of Satovar, a climbing plant of India, can be mixed with honey, milk and clarified butter. This pleasant tasting combination increases the secretion of semen in the male and corrects many disorders of the female and male genitals.

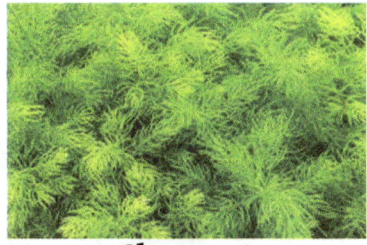

Shatovari

SPREADING HOGWEED

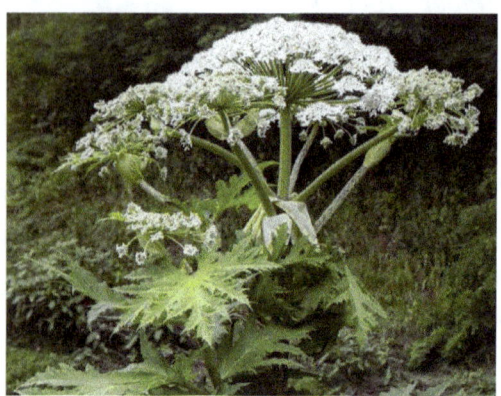

Hogweed

The root of another botanical from India, Spreading Hogweed, can be ground into a powder and applied to the soles of the feet to delay ejaculation. It will be remembered that elsewhere in this.book two other instances of this unusual method of application were cited—Henna and Sensitive plant. There are two kinds of Spreading Hogweed found in India: red and white. White is the one which is used.

GOTU KOLA

Gotu Kola is a member of the pennywort family closely related to Fo-ti-tieng. It is native to India, the nearby islands of India and parts of South Africa. In these places it is used as a blood purifier and brain energizer. A few fresh, raw leaves eaten daily will revitalize the brain and sex organs. It is also used to prevent nervous breakdown.

The Sinhalese have a saying about this herb: "Two leaves a day keep old age away." If the seeds are obtainable it can be grown in hot houses or outdoors in warm climates. The plant favors wet marshlands. If the fresh plant is not available, the dried leaves can be sprinkled on food or made as a tea.

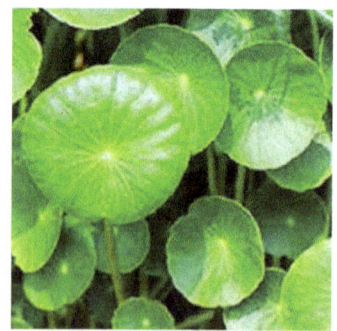

Gotu Kola

KINGO ROOT

(Geranium maculatum)

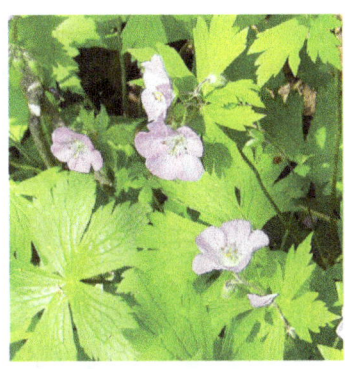

Kingo root—Wild Alum

Another astringent herb which is used as a douche before intercourse to tighten the vagina is Kingo root, also known as wild alum. The broken root pieces can be boiled as a tea for this purpose and used again several times. Or one level teaspoon of the powder can be disolved in 1 pint of boiled water. Allow to cool before using.

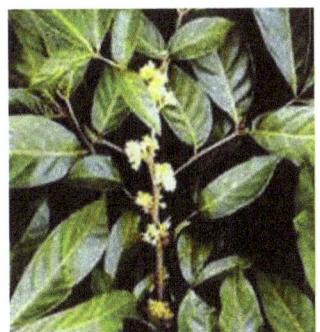

Muira Puama Bark

MUIRA PUAMA BARK

Muirapuama bark is chewed or boiled as a tea by natives of the Amazon and Orinoca basins in South America. It contains a resin which has strong stimulant and aphrodisiac qualities. Six to ten teaspoons are boiled for 15 minutes in one pint of water. I find it unpleasant to chew the bark because the wood splinters tend to catch in the throat. Some people smoke the bark for a stimulating high, but I find the smoke excessively harsh. The tea, however, is pleasant enough.

GUAIAC

Another exotic stimulant is Guaiac Bark from South America and the West Indies. Its

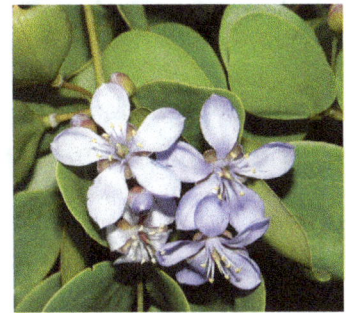

Guaiacum

active constituant is the resin. One ounce of the shavings
is boiled 15 minutes in one pint of water. One tablespoon
of this liquid is taken three times a day. It is often used in
combination with sarsaparilla as a blood purifier.

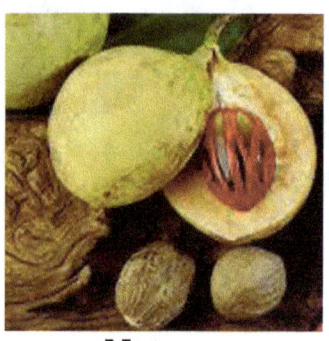

Nutmeg

NUTMEG

In Arabia Yemenite men consume large amounts of nutmeg
to increase virility. I would not
recommend more than a level
teaspoon at a time, because more
than that is likely to make a
person feel sluggish rather than
stimulated.

GINGER

Ginger is an invigorating stimulant for the gonads as well
as the body in general. The dried root or root powder
can be boiled as a tea with a dash of cloves and nutmeg
thrown in to improve
flavor.

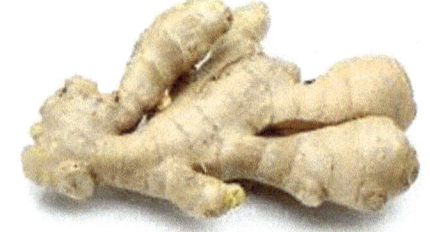

Ginger Root

It is most powerful,
however, when the fresh
root is chewed. It seems
hot to the taste, but does
no damage to the mucous
membranes. I have found
that chewing a few small pieces of the fresh root—an old
Chinese cure—will wipe out an oncoming cold or case of
flu in less than 30 minutes if used immediately at the first
symptoms.

VILCA

(Anadenanthera colubrina)

The Callahuayos of Boliv-
ia boil the seeds of vilca
(*Anadenanthera colubrina*)
in honey and water and
use it as a stimulant and
aphrodisiac.Vilca seeds are
also used as a powerful and
intoxicating snuff. I doubt if
the seeds can be easily pro-
cured in our own country.

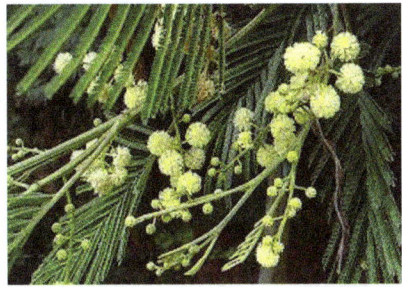

Anadenanthera Colubrina

SPICES AND CONDIMENTS

There is a long list of condiments and spices that have
had an impressive history as erotic stimulants especially
among the ancient Greeks and Romans. These include
anise, thyme, marioram. basil, rosemary, sage, savory, bay
leaf, celandine, myrrh, cinnamon alspice, benzoin, and
calamus. The stimulating effect of most of these spices
would probably be felt only by a person who has been for
some time on a bland diet.

Regular use of well seasoned foods inures us to most
of these mild stimulants.
Calamus is a different
matter, however. Asarone,
the essential oil of Acorus
calamus—also called
sweet flag root—contains
substantial quantities of
TMA-2, a substanceclose-
ly related to mescaline
and 18 times as potent.

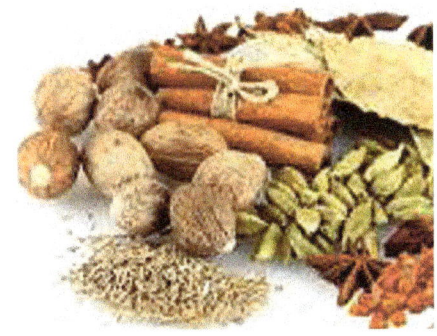

Sexy Spices & Condiments

APHRODISIACS

SUBSTANCES THAT ARE A TURN OFF

LADY'S SMOCK

(Cardamine pratensis)

Some people, especially those of earlier generations, who were uncomfortable with sexuality required medicines to

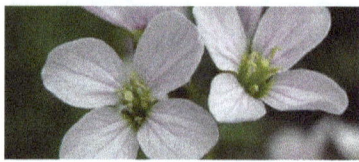

Lady's Smock

subdue their erotic urges rather than transgress their inhibiting puritanism by finding normal outlets for their needs. For them herbal doctors have prescribed wineglass doses of either Lady's Smock or Pussy willow 1 oz. per pint boiling water.

On the other hand many of us are unwittingly consuming substances that have a destructive effect on our sexual health. Lunch meats such as liverwurst, bologna, pastrami and hot dogs contain large amounts of potassium nitrate—saltpeter. This chemical was frequently sprinkled on prisoner's food to stifle sexual desire. Devital-

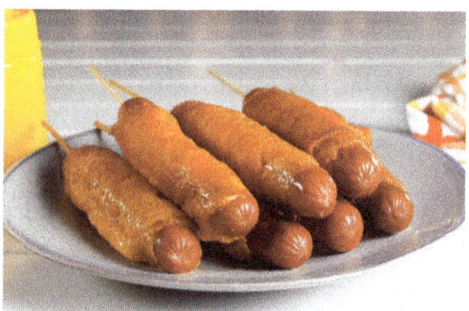

Hot dogs contain potassium nitrate—saltpeter

ized foods like these displace nutrient foods in our bodies and weaken our potency and general health.

Tobacco depletes our erotic powers, and—as everyone knows—kissing a person who smokes is like kissing an ashtray. Birth control pills upset the normal hormone balance in women and frequently cause loss of libido and frigidity.

Toxic preservatives and chemical additives help to make women frigid and turn men into sexual weaklings. Because it relaxes our inhibitions a little alcohol—preferably white wine—can sharpen Cupid's arrow, but even a little too much can dull it.

COFFEE

A cup of coffee on occasion may give us a lift and possible waken sexual vigor during a moment of laziness, but excessive and habitual coffee drinking definitely weakens sexuality.

Other offenders are aspirin compounds, menthol, and too frequent use of citrus fruit—especially limes, acid drinks, vinegar, verbain and valerian.

COCA BUSH

(Erythroxylum coca)

Many people find cocaine a wonderful aphrodisiac and I have found no indications of harm in the moderate use of this illegal substance. A popular thrill in South American countries where the coca bush grows is to rub the penis with coca leaves before intercourse. This delays ejaculation, creates the illusion—for the male—that his organ is gigantic and increases the intensity of orgasm.

A dab of cocaine on the head of the penis gives a

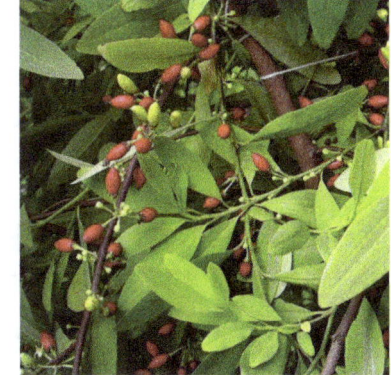

Coca Bush

man great staying power. On the clitoris it heightens a woman's pleasure. Excess snuffing of cocaine destroys the olefactory nerves—sense of smell—and may ultimately weaken sexuality.

APHRODISIAC FOODS

PRICKLY ASPARAGUS

Culpepper, one of the most respected of the early herbalists once wrote of prickly asparagus: "A decoction of the roots boiled in wine being taken fasting several mornings together stirreth up bodily lust in a man or women whatever some hath written to the contrary".

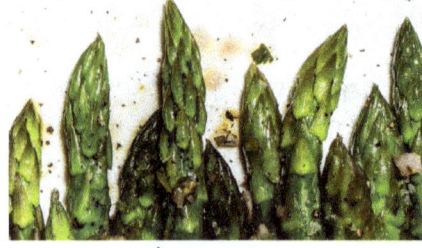

Asparagus

Folklore and a multitude of herbalists confirm this statement and hold that the use of either the roots, stalks or seeds is effective. Several modern authorities have expressed their doubts about the plant's usefulness as a love stimulant and insist that the phallic appearance of the shoots were the sole foundation for any such claims. I have found a scientific basis for the vegetable's salacious reputation, however, may permanently end this dispute.

The metabolism of protein in our bodies produces excess amounts of ammonia that linger in our tissues and make us tired, sluggish, irritable and sexual uninterested. Asparagus contains substantial quantities of aspartic acid, an amino acid which neutralizes and removes these waste products. Experiments with potassium and magnesium salts of aspartic acid have overcome cases of chronic exhaustion and increased sexual responsiveness in a matter of days. Asparagus is also rich in potassium, phosphorus and calcium, all necessary for maintenance of a high energy level. Soybeans and beets are also abundant in aspartic acid. Beets have a reputation as an aphrodisiac food dating back to Greek and Roman times.

GARLIC

Garlic, the delicious little bulb whose odor has a reputation for driving away vampires—as well as nearly everyone else—has many aphrodisiac qualities for the one who has eaten it if not for the one who has to kiss the one who eats it. If grown in the proper soil it contains adequate amounts of iodine necessary to healthy thyroid function.

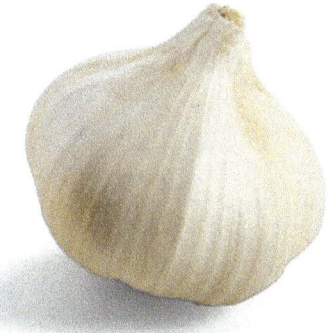

Garlic

In India men rub a mixture of garlic and lard on the penis and back to secure a powerful erection. The Ammites of China, one of the most lascivious peoples in the world, credit much of their lustiness to the large quantities of garlic they consume.

PUMPKIN SEEDS

Throughout Eastern Europe the Gypsies use large portions of raw pumpkin seeds as a food and recognize that this prevents prostrate disorders and preserves male potency. The raw seeds contain hormones that are good for the genito-urinary passages and promote male hormone production.

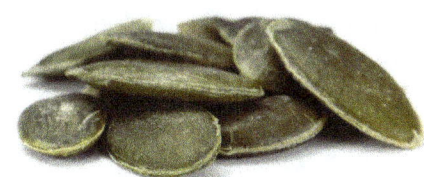

Pumpkin Seeds

They are also a rich source of phosphorus, B vitamins
and unsaturated fatty acids. All of these nutriments, as we
shall explain later, are essential for a healthy sex life.

COCOA

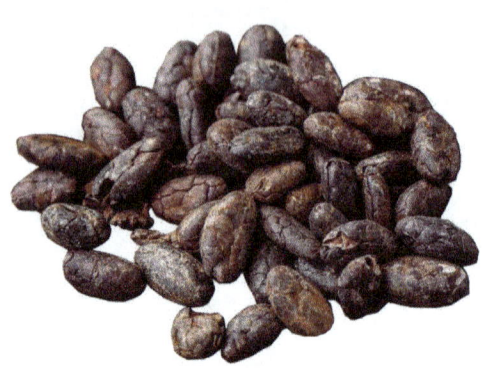

Cocoa Beans

Men working in
chocolate factories
and drinking cocoa
and milk to near
excess have reported
a notable increase
in sex drive. This
may be due to the
stimulating alkaloid,
theobromine found
in that beverage.
hocolate as a love
potion, however. Too
much coca robs the body of calcium and tends to clog the
kidneys. Also, the large amounts of sweetener—natural
or synthetic—taken with the drink are not good for our
bodies.

HONEY

Honey has been creditted with aphrodisiac properties. But
this discovery was made in the earlier ages before large,
commercial enterprises started refining it and adulterat-
ing it with sugar or corn syrup. If you use honey, buy the
dark, unclarified kind from a repuable health food store.
Actually the sexual and nutritional qualities of honey are
due to the presence of pollen granules. Pollen is a food we
are not used to. It is delicious plain or sprinkled on des-
serts or in milk shakes. It is high in protein, vitamin C, B
vitamins and minerals. It also contains substances which
stimulate the production of sex hormones.

Erotic stimulation has been attributed to many foods. We will present a list at the end of this section. Often the potency of these victuals has been greatly exaggerated. Nevertheless there is a definite connection between nutrition and healthy sexual function. The stimulating effect of certain foods, condiments and herbs depends greatly upon what the body is accustomed to. For example: if a person who has been a strict vegetarian for a long time were to eat a large rare steak, he or she would feel a tremendous rush of blood pressure within 15 minutes, his face would become flushed, his body warm and his or her sexual urges would be most intense.

After a few more similar dinners, however, he or she would become accustomed to the stimulating substances in meat and these reactions would no longer be so pronounced.

OTHER APHRODISIAC FOODS

Fish,
Shellfish
   esp oysters,
Caviar,
Shad roe,
Cod-liver oil,
Wild game,
Liver,
Kidneys,
Tripe,
Animal testes,
Lobsters,
Crabs,
Crayfish,
Shrimp,
Milk,

Eggs,
Carrots,
Turnips,
Artichokes,
Legumes,
Radishes,
Horseradish,
Paprika,
Mustard,
Saffron,
Gentian,
Chia seeds,
Curry,
Cardamoms,
Figs,

Fresh fruit
   esp - grapes
   and cherries
   but not too
   much citrus),
Yeast products,
Mushrooms
Tuffles.

SEX AND NUTRITION

Now that we have begun to understand the influence of vitamins, minerals and other nutriments on general health more people are taking a positive and active interest in seeing that they and their families are provided correctly with all of these necessities. This is not a fad; it is common sense.

We know how detrimental it would be if we should fail to supply our automobiles with the correct oil, water and gasoline. It is even more important with our bodies, which are living machines with specific needs that we must understand. We should not treat them badly or feed them junk. Unlike our cars we can not trade them in for new ones when they break down.

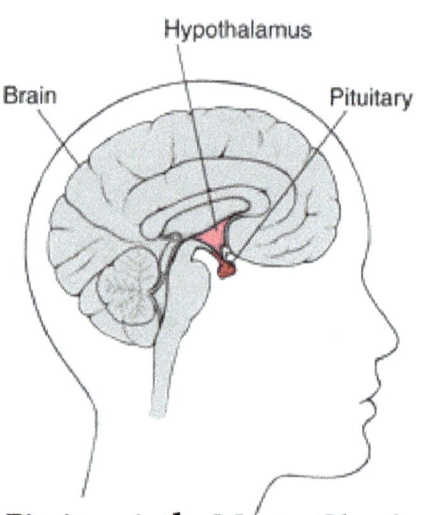

Pituitary is the Master Gland

General health influences sexual health, of course. The condition of our nerves, blood, arteries, heart, muscle tone and digestion can greatly determine our abilities in bed. Our sexuality is not merely in our gonads. It permiates every cell in our bodies. One of the farthest organs from the genitals is the pituitary gland. It lies at the base of the brain and has more to do with our sexuality than any other single organ in the body. It is often called the master gland because it produces hormones that in turn influence the hormone production of all other glands.

It is divided into two sections: the anterior pituitary and the posterior pituitary. Generally speaking the anterior influences male sexual activity—sex hormone and sperm production and masculine personality traits—while the posterior influences female activity—sex hormone and milk production, uterine contractions during labor and feminine personality traits.

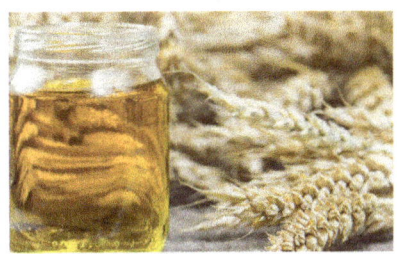

Wheat Germ Oil is high in Vitamin E.

Also, this double sided gland prevents premature aging of the sexual organs and early menopause. These remarks are a simplified description of pituitary activities. It is infinitely more complex. To function properly this gland requires ample protein, B vitamins—especially B2, pantothenic acid and choline—and vitamin E. The latter, which is often called the sex vitamin, is found in greater concentration in the pituitary than anywhere else in the body. It particularly effects the anterior pituitary's influence on male hormone production.

This is one reason why men who have been taking large doses of vitamin E or wheat germ oil usually notice a marked increase in their sexual capacities. The antioxydent nature of this vitamin helps to retard the aging process. It also protects the sex hormones from oxydizing. Extreme deficiency of vitamin E can lead to wasting diseases, weakness of the muscle tissues, disorders of the reproductive glands, incurable degeneration of the testes, sterility, miscarriage, stillbirths, and spontaneous abortion. Vitamin E has been used successfully to treat difficult menopause symptoms; hot flashes, backache, excess menstrual flow, high blood pressure and muscle pains. It also improves heart response.

This is an advantage for athletes of both the outdoor and "indoor" variety. Since it is non-toxic 400 to 1600 units or more can be taken daily without any ill effects.

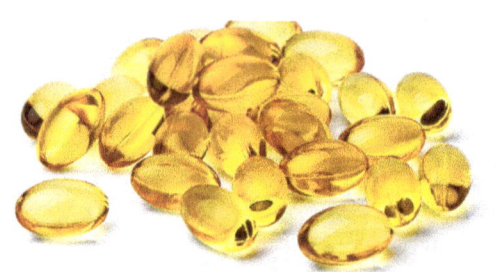

Daily use of cod-live-oil boosts sex drive

The only circumstances under which large amounts of the vitamin might be unadvisable are where the person is already receiving insulin, digitalis or heavy doses of iron. Vitamin E is found in raw, unrefined vegetable oils unroasted seeds and nuts, and raw wheat germ. If you buy the vitamin itself get 400 unit capsules of natural mixed tocopherols. Synthetic vitamin E requires six times the natural dosage to approximate the same results.

Vitamin A works hand in hand with vitamin E. If you are using lots of E you should also get 25,000 units of A. Unsaturated fatty acids—sometimes called vitamin F—are necessary for the proper assimilation of A and E. They are required for normal gland activity and have been used to treat prostate and menstrual disorders. They are found in raw oils along with E. Abundant use of vitamin F increases sexual potency. .

Daily use of cod-liver oil has been found to augment the sex drive. It is rich in vitamins A and D. The latter has a way of energizing the body at the same time as relaxing it. The hormones of the adrenal and prostate glands are extremely rich in vitamin C so we must keep them well supplied with this substance. Besides its many other uses in protecting us from colds and spinal problems, this vitamin also prevents varicose veins in pregnant women. Combined with B complex vitamins it helps to regulate the flow of female sex hormones. Although the National Research Council—the government agency which sets the minimum daily requirements—tells us that 30mg per day is sufficient, this amount for most people is barely enough to prevent scurvy, which is the final stage of C deficiency. Actually most of us should take about 3,000 mg daily—1,000 with each meal.

All of the B complex vitamins influence the production of sex hormones in both the male and female; all are necessary for general health. Some of the B vitamins have very specific effects on sexual health and bedroom ability. Bl is required to convert body fuels into energy. Deficiency soon results fatigue, depression, anxiety and apathy. B2, the youth vitamin, keeps the skin lustrous and alive. B3, niacin, overcomes schizophrenic tendencies which no one wants in a lover. Choline keeps the arteries young. Biotin preserves mental health and appetite. And B12 helps to control degeneration of the central nervous system. Deficience of this vitamin in men results in sterility.

In women during the embrionic stage of pregnancy B12 deficiency may deform the child with hair-lip, clefpalate or blindness. Another important B vitamin of which you may never have heard is vitamin B15—pangamic acid. Its function is to bring oxygen, the supporter of life, to all the tissues. Because of this it helps to prevent premature impotence, and most degenerative diseases including old age. Rats that were given large doses of B15 had extended periods of youth and nearly doubled their life span. The reason you may never have heard of it is because information has been suppressed. Vitamin B15 is illegal in this country. You can not even get it on prescription. It is used freely and with much success in many other countries including the Soviet Union.

Why has the Food Drug Administration forbidden Americans to use it? They explain that it has not been properly tested, but have made no attempts to test it themselves. They say that it may

All of the B complex vitamins influence the production of sex hormones in both the male and female; all are necessary for general health.

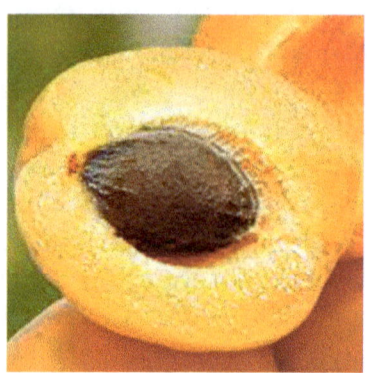

Apricot kernal is a rich source of Vit B15.

have some toxic side effects. Yet the toxic dose is 10,000 times the therapeutic dose. Compare this to the toxic dose of aspirin of any of the nonprescription cold medicines—none of which do any good. If you love the American Medical Association you had best avoid this vitamin. Think of how much money—and power—they will lose if the incidence of arterial sclerosis, heart disease and cancer in the United States is vastly reduced.

If you seek a long, healthy and sexually active life you will have to get the forbidden vitamin from natural sources. Yeast products are quite good, but by far the richest source of vitamin B15 is the kernel of the apricot. These little almond-like nuts are a favorite food of the Hunzas, those incredibly healthy people of the Himalayas who have no doctors and usually live to be well over a hundred. There is more in the apricot kernel than vitamin B15, but we will talk about that later in this book.

Deficiency in iron results in tired blood. An anemic person is almost bound to be a failure in bed. Iron is best absorbed from natural food sources along with vitamin C. It is found abundantly in most vegetables, fruits and meats, and is especially plentiful in liver and yeast. The main proble,m with iron is that it is difficult for some people to absorb it into their system. An apple eaten after a meal tremendously assists the absorbtion of iron. Potassium, magnesium and calcium are important in bur sex lives because they help to overcome exhaustion. Manganese is important in reproduction and the proper function of the mammary gjands.

Zinc plays a significant roll in the growth and maturity of the male sexual organs. Deficiency results in unhealthy changes in the structure and size of the prostate gland. There is more zinc in the male reproductive system than anywhere else in the body. The highest concentration is in the prostate and seminal fluids and most of all in the sperm cells. More than 60% of America's soil is deficient in zinc. Artificial fertilizers are largely to blame.Some of the best sources are nuts, seeds (especially pumpkin, sunflower and sesame seeds), liver and yeast.

There is a larger proportion of lecithin in the brain, central nervous system and seminal fluids than in any other part of the body. It must be replaced after orgasm-Good sources are unrefined vegetable oils, unroasted seeds or nuts, and eggs. German physicians are now using lecithin tablets to treat neurasthenia resulting from sexual debility.

Protein starvation is the most prevalent form of malnutrition in the world today. Yet protein is found in nearly all the natural foods we eat. The problem is that protein is composed of amino acids. Many ot these we can form in our bodies from other amino acids, but eight of them we can not construct so it is essential that we get them from food. All eight are found together in meat, fish, fowl, eggs and dairy products. If you are a vegetarian you must get plenty of soybeans—one of the few vegetables which have all eight—or else know how to combine your foods so that one supplements what is lacking in the other.

One of the eight essential amino acids, Arginine is especially important in our sex lives. It comprises 80% of the sperm cells. A deficiency leads to loss of sexual instinct

Sperm cells are made of 80% Arginine.

in both men and women. In males it may result in impotence, sterility, and decrease in production and mobility of sperm cells. Tryptophane, also one of the eight, if lacking can prevent women from conceiving and may cause testicle degeneration in the male. Deficient lysine can also lead to reproductive problems.

All this talk about nutrition, health and sex may not seem important to many while young when they have abundances of sexual energy. But what we do now determines how things will be later. A little wisdom put to practice can protect us against decline in the future and add more zest to our love lives during the present.

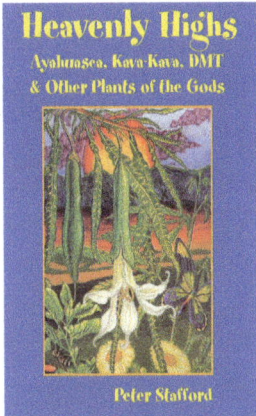
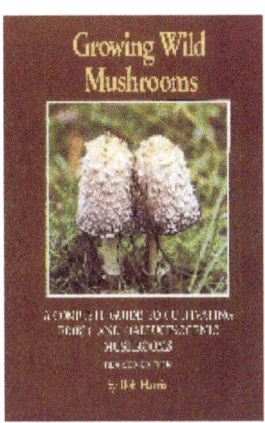
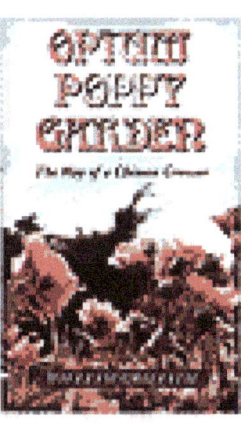
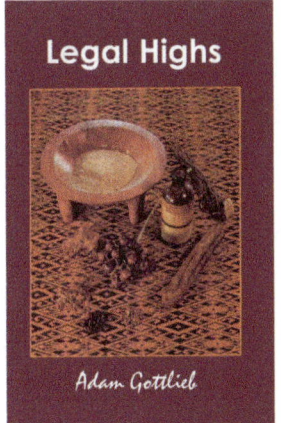
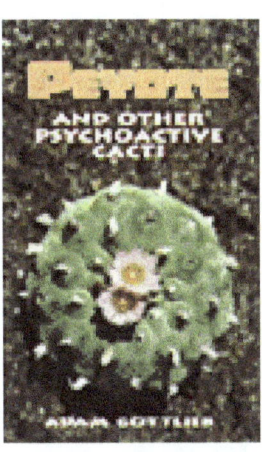
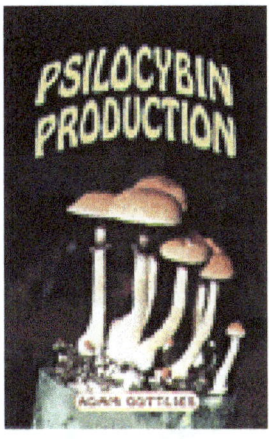